LOW CARB DIET COOKBOOK FOR ENDOMORPS

High Protein Recipes and Meal Plan for Endomorphs to do Low-Carb Better and More Deliciously

Dr. Ella J Carpender

Copyright © 2024

All Rights Are Reserved

The content in this book may not be reproduced, duplicated, or transferred without the express written permission of the author or publisher. Under no circumstances will the publisher or author be held liable or legally responsible for any losses, expenditures, or damages incurred directly or indirectly as a consequence of the information included in this book.

Legal Remarks

Copyright protection applies to this publication. It is only intended for personal use. No piece of this work may be modified, distributed, sold, quoted, or paraphrased without the author's or publisher's consent.

Disclaimer Statement

Please keep in mind that the contents of this booklet are meant for educational and recreational purposes. Every effort has been made to offer accurate, up-to-date, reliable, and thorough information. There are, however, no stated or implied assurances of any kind. Readers understand that the author is providing competent counsel. The content in this book originates from several sources. Please seek the opinion of a competent professional before using any of the tactics outlined in this book. By reading this book, the reader agrees that the author will not be held accountable for any direct or indirect damages resulting from the use of the information contained therein, including, but not limited to, errors, omissions, or inaccuracies.

TABLE OF CONTENTS

INTRODUCTION

Understanding body types is crucial in tailoring nutrition and exercise programs to meet individual needs. The endomorph kind of body is usually identified as a body that tends to store fat more, has a wider bony structure, and often plagues the question of weight control. Affording this understanding is of particular importance, given that one goes about the discussions related to dietary approaches and, indeed, even the efficacy of low-carb eating with regards to the endomorph body type.

With a slow metabolism, therefore, it's quite hard for endomorphs to lose weight, and they become easy gainers. Endomorph body types have a tendency for fat storage in the lower regions of the body, hence a pear shape. Despite all the above, endomorphs can still control their weight and improve their health with the right dietary strategy. This is where low-carb eating comes in to offer a workable solution to the metabolic hiccups of the endomorphs.

The science of the low-carb diet for endomorphs really depends on how their bodies metabolize carbohydrates. Carbohydrates form the major energy source for the body, breaking down to glucose and later consumed as energy or stored as glycogen in muscles and the liver. When it is more than the glycogen reservoir can fill, then any extra glucose is stored as fat. With this efficient conversion of glucose to fat, endomorphs have to be very precise with their level of carbohydrate intake, since the rate at which it is metabolized is so slow.

The low-carb regime limits the amount of carbohydrate intake; therefore, there is little fuel for energy. It makes the body turn to stored fats in order to get energy and therefore leads to the process called ketosis. This methodology of diet may bring about endomorphs being able to control insulin spikes, moderating blood sugar levels, and, indirectly, weight control and management of health. They should observe a diet with high-quality proteins, good fats, and vegetables low in carbohydrates, all of which would make their bodies get the maximum support of metabolism for their muscles.

But this does not mean that they should reduce carbs; one should focus on the quality of the consumed carbohydrate, of course. Most endomorphs benefit from the intake of complex carbohydrates with a low glycemic index, such as leafy greens, non-starchy veggies, and whole grains in moderation. This type of carb also provides energy, but without the huge peaks of insulin characterizing simple sugars found in sweets, white bread, and other types of junk food.

A low-carb diet could require pretty high knowledge of the right foodstuffs and amounts. Endomorphs should try to ensure that the plate is covered with lean proteins, good fats, and a lot of low-carb veggies. This balance is not just to maintain weight but, in the same way, for healthy nutrients not to be ingested in the right quantities by the body. Some fiber-rich foods such as avocados, nuts, seeds, and berries can also help with satiety in preventing overeating.

Another vital aspect of managing endomorph body type is exercise. Evidently, diet counts for a lot when it comes to weight management; this can be better enhanced by following up a low carbohydrate eating plan and having a consistent exercise routine. Strength training is also very good for endomorphs, as it will increase lean mass and also, in doing so, increase metabolic rate, therefore improving fat-burning potential.

Cardiovascular exercise, more precisely high-intensity interval training (HIIT), is also very efficient in fat burning and helps improve overall cardiovascular health. Right exercise routine followed by endomorphs also includes united dietary change for proper management of body type leading to sustainable weight loss and well-being.

The important thing for endomorphs to remember is that, while having many benefits, low-carb eating doesn't keep absolute measures. One should always remember that one's own responses to carbohydrate restriction can be very individual, and what works for one person may not be tolerated in the same manner by another. Thus, it is very important to listen to your body, and modify different approaches to your diet as necessary. Seeking counsel from an instructive health provider or a registered dietitian may offer an approach to personal advice concerning living the low-carb way of life.

THE BASICS OF LOW CARB EATING

What Are Carbohydrates?

Carbohydrates are one of the three macronutrients, alongside proteins and fats, that are essential for our body's proper functioning. They are found in a wide range of foods and are the body's primary source of energy. Carbohydrates are classified into three main types: sugars, starches, and fibre. Sugars are simple carbohydrates, consisting of one or two molecules, and are found in foods like fruits, vegetables, milk, and sweetened products. Starches are complex carbohydrates, made up of many sugar molecules linked together, and are present in grains, legumes, and root vegetables. Fiber, also a complex carbohydrate, is unique because the human body cannot digest it, yet it plays a crucial role in maintaining digestive health.

Understanding the role of carbohydrates is crucial, especially for endomorphs, who tend to have a slower metabolism and a higher propensity to store fat. This knowledge becomes a powerful tool when applied to dietary choices, particularly the adoption of a low carb eating plan. Low carb diets focus on reducing the intake of carbohydrates, especially those that are quickly digested and cause spikes in blood sugar levels. Instead, these diets emphasize foods high in protein and fat, along with low-carb vegetables.

The Benefits of Low Carb Eating for Endomorphs

By reducing carbohydrate intake, endomorphs can better manage their insulin levels. Insulin is a hormone that regulates blood sugar levels and plays a key role in fat storage. High carbohydrate meals cause a rapid increase in blood sugar, leading to spikes in insulin. Over time, this can lead to insulin resistance, a condition where the body's cells become less responsive to insulin, making it harder to manage weight. A low carb diet helps mitigate these spikes, improving insulin sensitivity and making it easier for the body to use stored fat as energy.

Moreover, low carb eating can lead to an automatic reduction in calorie intake. Foods high in protein and fat are more satiating, helping to reduce hunger and the overall amount of food consumed. This can create a natural calorie deficit, which is essential for weight loss. Additionally, by limiting carbohydrate intake, endomorphs can shift their body's reliance from carbs to fats as a primary energy source, a process known as ketosis. This metabolic state can lead to increased fat burning, further supporting weight loss efforts.

Another benefit of low carb eating for endomorphs is the potential for improved heart health. Diets low in carbohydrates and high in healthy fats can lead to reductions in blood triglycerides, a type of fat found in the blood, and increases in high-density lipoprotein (HDL) cholesterol, often referred to as "good" cholesterol. These changes can help lower the risk of heart disease.

How to Calculate Your Carb Intake

The amount of carbohydrates an individual needs can vary based on several factors, including age, sex, body composition, activity level, and personal health goals. For endomorphs aiming to lose weight, a common recommendation is to start with a daily intake of 100 to 150 grams of carbohydrates. This range is considered low carb but not so restrictive that it becomes difficult to maintain long-term.

To calculate your specific carb intake, begin by determining your daily calorie needs. This can be done using an online calculator or by consulting with a healthcare professional. Once you know how many calories you need, you can allocate a percentage of those calories to carbohydrates. For a low carb diet, carbohydrates might make up 20% to 30% of your total daily calories. For example, if you're consuming 2,000 calories a day, 400 to 600 of those calories could come from carbohydrates. Since each gram of carbohydrate provides 4 calories, this translates to 100 to 150 grams of carbohydrates per day.

It's also important to focus on the quality of the carbohydrates you consume. Opt for nutrient-dense, whole foods like vegetables, fruits, and whole grains, and limit the intake of refined carbs and sugars. These healthier options have a lower glycaemic index, meaning they have a slower, smaller impact on blood sugar levels.

PREPARING YOUR KITCHEN

Making the transition to a low-carb lifestyle, particularly for those with an endomorph body type, calls for more than dietary adjustments. It calls for a change of perspective when it comes to cooking and food preparation. The kitchen, the centre of the house, is where this makeover starts. Foundational steps in this path include preparing your kitchen with necessary appliances, filling your fridge and pantry with appropriate ingredients, and learning how to read food labels to determine the amount of carbohydrates.

Essential Kitchen Tools

Creating delicious and nutritious low-carb meals is an art and science that requires the right tools. These tools not only make meal preparation easier but also more enjoyable. A well-equipped kitchen should have a set of high-quality knives, including a chef's knife, a paring knife, and a serrated knife. These are indispensable for chopping vegetables, fruits, and meats with precision and ease. A set of cutting boards, preferably in different colours to prevent cross-contamination between raw meats and vegetables, is also essential.

In addition to knives and cutting boards, a variety of pots and pans are necessary for cooking a wide range of dishes. A non-stick skillet is ideal for frying and sautéing, while a large stockpot is perfect for soups and stews. A cast-iron skillet can be a versatile addition, suitable for everything from searing meats to baking low-carb bread. Baking sheets and silicone baking mats are also crucial for roasting vegetables and baking low-carb treats.

Small kitchen appliances can further simplify the low-carb cooking process. A food processor is a versatile tool that can be used for chopping vegetables, making cauliflower rice, or preparing homemade nut butters. A blender is essential for smoothies and soups, and a slow cooker or an instant pot can make meal preparation effortless, allowing for healthy meals to be ready with minimal hands-on time.

Stocking Your Pantry and Fridge

The key to sustaining a low-carb lifestyle lies in having a well-stocked pantry and fridge. This ensures that you have the necessary ingredients on hand to whip up low-carb meals and snacks without resorting to high-carb options. Your pantry should include a variety of spices and herbs to add flavor to dishes without adding carbs. Stock up on olive oil, coconut oil, and avocado oil, which are healthy fats ideal for cooking and dressing salads.

Low-carb staples such as almond flour, coconut flour, and flaxseed meal are essential for baking and breading. Nuts and seeds, along with their butters, are great for snacks and adding texture to meals. Canned goods like tomatoes, olives, and coconut milk can be lifesavers for quick meals. Don't forget to include low-carb sweeteners, such as stevia or erythritol, for when you need a touch of sweetness without the carbs.

In the fridge, prioritize fresh vegetables, especially leafy greens and low-carb options like broccoli, cauliflower, and zucchini. Eggs, high-quality meats, and fatty fish should also have a place in your refrigerator, providing you with essential proteins and fats. Cheese, butter, and full-fat dairy (in moderation) can add richness and flavor to your dishes. Avocados, berries, and lemons or limes are also great to have on hand for their nutritional value and ability to enhance the taste of meals.

Reading Food Labels for Carb Content

Understanding how to read food labels is crucial for maintaining a low-carb diet. Food labels provide valuable information about the nutritional content of food items, allowing you to make informed choices about what to include in your diet. When reading food labels, focus on the total carbohydrate content, which includes sugars, starches, and fibre. However, since fibre does not raise blood sugar levels the way other carbohydrates do, you can subtract the fibre content from the total carbs to calculate the net carbs, which is a more accurate reflection of a food's impact on your blood sugar.

Pay attention to the serving size listed on the label, as all the nutritional information provided is based on this amount. It's easy to underestimate how many servings you're actually consuming, which can lead to unintentional carb intake. Also, be wary of terms like "sugar-free" or "low-carb," as these products can still contain carbs in the form of sugar alcohols or other ingredients. Always check the ingredient list for hidden sources of carbs, such as added sugars, starches, and fillers.

BEYOND THE DIET

Achieving and sustaining optimal health requires incorporating exercise into one's lifestyle, particularly for those with an endomorph body type. An organised fitness programme is especially beneficial for endomorphs, who tend to acquire weight more easily and have a higher percentage of body fat. This programme helps with weight management as well as improving overall health, muscle mass, and metabolic health.

Incorporating Exercise

For endomorphs, the integration of exercise into daily life is crucial. The challenge often lies not in the act itself but in finding and maintaining the motivation and consistency required for long-term success. The key is to start slowly, setting realistic goals and gradually increasing the intensity and duration of workouts as fitness improves. Incorporating exercise doesn't mean dedicating hours at the gym daily; it can start with simple changes, such as taking the stairs instead of the elevator, going for a walk during lunch breaks, or engaging in short, high-intensity workouts at home.

Diversity in exercise types can prevent boredom and enhance motivation. A mix of cardiovascular exercises, strength training, and flexibility workouts can keep the routine interesting and cover all aspects of fitness. Additionally, finding a workout buddy or joining a fitness community can provide the necessary encouragement and accountability to stay on track.

Best Exercises for Endomorphs

Endomorphs benefit most from exercises that maximize calorie burn, enhance muscle mass, and improve insulin sensitivity. A combination of high-intensity interval training (HIIT), strength training, and steady-state cardio can yield significant benefits.

HIIT involves short bursts of intense activity followed by brief rest periods. This type of workout is highly effective for endomorphs as it boosts metabolism and increases fat burning, even after the exercise session has ended. HIIT can be applied to various activities, including sprinting, biking, jump rope, or bodyweight exercises, making it a versatile option that can be tailored to individual preferences and fitness levels.

Strength training is another crucial component of an endomorph's exercise regimen. By building lean muscle mass, endomorphs can increase their resting metabolic rate, as muscle tissue burns more calories than fat tissue, even at rest. Focusing on compound movements such as squats, deadlifts, bench presses, and rows can engage multiple muscle groups, leading to more efficient workouts. Incorporating bodyweight exercises, resistance bands, free weights, or machines can add variety and challenge the muscles in different ways.

Steady-state cardio, such as walking, jogging, swimming, or cycling, should also be part of an endomorph's exercise plan. While not as intense as HIIT, steady-state cardio can be an effective way to burn calories and improve cardiovascular health. It's particularly useful for those who may not be ready to engage in high-intensity workouts or as a way to add low-impact exercise on recovery days.

Creating a Balanced Workout Routine

A balanced workout routine for endomorphs should address cardiovascular health, muscle building, and flexibility. An effective strategy is to alternate between different types of workouts throughout the week, allowing for adequate recovery time between intense sessions.

A sample weekly plan might include two to three days of strength training, focusing on different muscle groups each day to allow for muscle recovery. Two days of HIIT, lasting 20 to 30 minutes per session, can provide significant metabolic benefits without the risk of overtraining. One to two days of steady-state cardio can add variety and enhance endurance. Incorporating at least one day of flexibility training, such as yoga or Pilates, can improve mobility, reduce the risk of injury, and offer a restorative element to the exercise regimen.

Rest and recovery are as important as the workouts themselves. Endomorphs should ensure they are allowing their bodies to recover adequately to prevent burnout and injuries. This includes getting enough sleep, staying hydrated, and incorporating active recovery days where exercise is more about movement and less about intensity.

BREAKFAST RECIPES

Almond Flour Pancakes

Ingredients:

- 1 cup almond flour
- 3 large eggs, ¼ cup water
- 1 tbsp coconut oil, melted
- 2 tsp erythritol (or sweetener of choice)
- 1 tsp baking powder, ½ tsp vanilla extract
- Pinch of salt
- Butter or oil for cooking

Prep Time: 10 mins

Cooking Time: 15 mins

Total Time: 25 mins

Servings: 2

Nutrition Facts (per serving):

- Calories: 345
- Fat: 29g
- Saturated Fat: 8g
- Cholesterol: 279mg
- Sodium: 136mg
- Carbohydrate: 11g
- Fiber: 6g
- Protein: 15g

Directions:

1. In a mixing bowl, whisk together the almond flour, eggs, water, melted coconut oil, erythritol, baking powder, vanilla extract, and a pinch of salt until smooth.

2. Heat a non-stick skillet over medium heat and brush with a little butter or oil.

3. Pour ¼ cup of batter for each pancake onto the skillet. Cook until bubbles form on the surface, then flip and cook until golden brown on the other side, about 2-3 minutes per side.

4. Serve warm with your choice of low-carb toppings, such as berries or sugar-free syrup.

Spinach and Feta Omelette

Ingredients:

- 3 large eggs
- 1 cup fresh spinach, chopped
- ¼ cup feta cheese, crumbled
- 2 tbsp olive oil
- Salt and pepper to taste

Prep Time: 5 mins

Cooking Time: 10 mins

Total Time: 15 mins

Servings: 1

Nutrition Facts (per serving):

- Calories: 400
- Fat: 34g
- Saturated Fat: 10g
- Cholesterol: 558mg
- Sodium: 682mg
- Carbohydrate: 4g
- Fiber: 1g
- Protein: 22g

Directions:

1. Beat the eggs in a bowl and season with salt and pepper.

2. Heat olive oil in a skillet over medium heat. Add the spinach and sauté until wilted, about 2 minutes.

3. Pour the beaten eggs over the spinach. Cook for a few minutes until the edges start to set.

4. Sprinkle feta cheese over half of the omelette. Fold the other half over the cheese and cook until the cheese is melted and the eggs are set.

5. Serve hot.

Low Carb Breakfast Burrito

Ingredients:

- 2 large eggs, beaten
- 1 large low-carb tortilla
- ¼ cup shredded cheddar cheese
- 2 tbsp salsa
- ¼ avocado, sliced
- 2 slices cooked bacon, crumbled
- Salt and pepper to taste
- 1 tbsp olive oil

Prep Time: 5 mins

Cooking Time: 10 mins

Total Time: 15 mins

Servings: 1

Nutrition Facts (per serving):

- Calories: 485
- Fat: 38g
- Saturated Fat: 12g

- Cholesterol: 379mg

- Sodium: 875mg

- Carbohydrate: 18g

- Fiber: 9g

- Protein: 22g

Directions:

1. Heat olive oil in a skillet over medium heat. Add the beaten eggs and scramble until fully cooked. Season with salt and pepper.

2. Warm the low-carb tortilla in a separate skillet or microwave.

3. Place the scrambled eggs in the center of the tortilla. Top with shredded cheese, salsa, avocado slices, and crumbled bacon.

4. Fold the tortilla to enclose the filling, forming a burrito.

5. Serve immediately.

Chia Seed Pudding

Ingredients:

- ¼ cup chia seeds

- 1 cup unsweetened almond milk

- 1 tbsp erythritol (or sweetener of choice)

- ½ tsp vanilla extract

- A pinch of salt

- Berries for topping (optional)

Prep Time: 5 mins (plus overnight soaking)

Cooking Time: 0 mins

Total Time: 5 mins (plus overnight soaking)

Servings: 2

Nutrition Facts (per serving):

- Calories: 150
- Fat: 9g
- Saturated Fat: 1g
- Cholesterol: 0mg
- Sodium: 91mg
- Carbohydrate: 13g
- Fiber: 10g
- Protein: 5g

Directions:

1. In a bowl, mix together chia seeds, almond milk, erythritol, vanilla extract, and a pinch of salt.
2. Cover and refrigerate overnight, or at least 6 hours, until it achieves a pudding-like consistency.
3. Stir the pudding well before serving. Add more almond milk if needed to adjust the consistency.
4. Serve with fresh berries on top, if desired.

Smoked Salmon and Avocado Salad

Ingredients:

- 2 cups mixed salad greens
- 4 oz smoked salmon
- ½ avocado, sliced
- 2 tbsp olive oil
- 1 tbsp lemon juice
- Salt and pepper to taste
- 1 tbsp capers (optional)

Prep Time: 10 mins

Cooking Time: 0 mins

__Total Time:__ 10 mins

__Servings:__ 1

__Nutrition Facts (per serving):__

- Calories: 380
- Fat: 31g
- Saturated Fat: 5g
- Cholesterol: 22mg
- Sodium: 667mg
- Carbohydrate: 9g
- Fiber: 7g
- Protein: 18g

__Directions:__

1. Arrange the mixed salad greens on a plate.
2. Top with smoked salmon slices and avocado.
3. In a small bowl, whisk together olive oil, lemon juice, salt, and pepper to make the dressing.
4. Drizzle the dressing over the salad and toss gently to combine.
5. Garnish with capers, if using, and serve immediately.

Coconut Flour Porridge

__Ingredients:__

- ¼ cup coconut flour
- 1 cup unsweetened almond milk
- 1 egg, beaten
- 1 tbsp erythritol (or sweetener of choice)
- ½ tsp cinnamon
- ¼ tsp vanilla extract

- Pinch of salt

Prep Time: 5 mins

Cooking Time: 5 mins

Total Time: 10 mins

Servings: 1

Nutrition Facts (per serving):

- Calories: 215

- Fat: 12g

- Saturated Fat: 8g

- Cholesterol: 164mg

- Sodium: 123mg

- Carbohydrate: 18g

- Fiber: 10g

- Protein: 9g

Directions:

1. In a small saucepan, whisk together the coconut flour and almond milk over medium heat until well combined.

2. Stir in the beaten egg, erythritol, cinnamon, vanilla extract, and a pinch of salt. Continue to cook, stirring constantly, until the mixture thickens to a porridge-like consistency.

3. Remove from heat and let it cool slightly. Serve warm.

Zucchini Hash Browns

Ingredients:

- 2 cups grated zucchini (water squeezed out)

- 1 large egg

- ¼ cup almond flour

- ½ tsp garlic powder

- Salt and pepper to taste

- 2 tbsp olive oil for frying

Prep Time: 10 mins

Cooking Time: 10 mins

Total Time: 20 mins

Servings: 2

Nutrition Facts (per serving):

- Calories: 230
- Fat: 19g
- Saturated Fat: 3g
- Cholesterol: 93mg
- Sodium: 58mg
- Carbohydrate: 8g
- Fiber: 3g
- Protein: 7g

Directions:

1. In a mixing bowl, combine grated zucchini, egg, almond flour, garlic powder, salt, and pepper. Mix well to form a batter.

2. Heat olive oil in a skillet over medium heat. Scoop ¼ cup portions of the zucchini mixture into the skillet, flattening them into hash brown shapes.

3. Fry until golden brown and crispy, about 4-5 minutes per side. Serve hot.

Avocado and Egg Breakfast Bowl

Ingredients:

- 1 avocado, halved and pitted
- 2 eggs
- Salt and pepper to taste

- 1 tbsp chopped chives
- 1 tbsp olive oil

Prep Time: 5 mins

Cooking Time: 15 mins

Total Time: 20 mins

Servings: 1

Nutrition Facts (per serving):

- Calories: 480
- Fat: 40g
- Saturated Fat: 7g
- Cholesterol: 372mg
- Sodium: 124mg
- Carbohydrate: 17g
- Fiber: 13g
- Protein: 16g

Directions:

1. Preheat the oven to 425°F (220°C). Scoop out a bit more flesh from the avocado halves to make room for the eggs.

2. Place the avocado halves in a baking dish, ensuring they don't tip over. Crack an egg into each avocado half. Season with salt and pepper.

3. Bake in the preheated oven until the eggs are cooked to your liking, about 12-15 minutes.

4. Drizzle with olive oil and sprinkle chopped chives on top before serving.

Greek Yogurt with Nuts and Berries

Ingredients:

- 1 cup full-fat Greek yogurt

- ¼ cup mixed berries (strawberries, blueberries, raspberries)
- 2 tbsp chopped nuts (almonds, walnuts)
- 1 tbsp chia seeds
- 1 tbsp erythritol (or sweetener of choice)

Prep Time: 5 mins

Cooking Time: 0 mins

Total Time: 5 mins

Servings: 1

Nutrition Facts (per serving):

- Calories: 310
- Fat: 18g
- Saturated Fat: 5g
- Cholesterol: 25mg
- Sodium: 65mg
- Carbohydrate: 18g
- Fiber: 5g
- Protein: 20g

Directions:

1. In a serving bowl, combine the Greek yogurt with erythritol (or your choice of sweetener).
2. Top the yogurt with mixed berries, chopped nuts, and chia seeds.
3. Serve immediately for a refreshing and filling breakfast.

Turkey and Spinach Scramble

Ingredients:

- 4 oz ground turkey
- 1 cup fresh spinach

- 2 large eggs
- 1 tbsp olive oil
- Salt and pepper to taste
- ¼ tsp paprika

Prep Time: 5 mins

Cooking Time: 10 mins

Total Time: 15 mins

Servings: 1

Nutrition Facts (per serving):

- Calories: 320
- Fat: 23g
- Saturated Fat: 5g
- Cholesterol: 372mg
- Sodium: 127mg
- Carbohydrate: 2g
- Fiber: 1g
- Protein: 27g

Directions:

1. Heat olive oil in a skillet over medium heat. Add the ground turkey, season with salt, pepper, and paprika. Cook until browned and no longer pink, breaking it into small pieces as it cooks.

2. Add the fresh spinach to the skillet and cook until wilted, about 2 minutes.

3. Beat the eggs in a bowl and pour them over the turkey and spinach mixture. Cook, stirring occasionally, until the eggs are set.

4. Serve hot, with additional seasoning if desired.

Broccoli and Cheddar Cheese Soup

Ingredients:

- 2 cups broccoli florets, chopped
- 1 cup chicken or vegetable broth
- 1 cup heavy cream
- 1 cup shredded sharp cheddar cheese
- 2 tbsp butter
- 1 small onion, diced
- 2 cloves garlic, minced
- Salt and pepper to taste
- ¼ tsp nutmeg

Prep Time: 10 mins

Cooking Time: 20 mins

Total Time: 30 mins

Servings: 2

Nutrition Facts (per serving):

- Calories: 495
- Fat: 44g
- Saturated Fat: 27g
- Cholesterol: 163mg
- Sodium: 807mg
- Carbohydrate: 10g
- Fiber: 2g
- Protein: 17g

Directions:

1. In a large pot, melt butter over medium heat. Add onion and garlic, sautéing until translucent.

2. Add broccoli and broth. Bring to a boil, then reduce heat and simmer until broccoli is tender, about 10 minutes.

3. Stir in heavy cream, cheddar cheese, nutmeg, salt, and pepper. Cook until the cheese is melted and the soup is heated through.

4. For a smoother soup, use an immersion blender to blend until desired consistency is reached.

5. Serve hot, garnished with extra cheese if desired.

Cauliflower Hash

Ingredients:

- 2 cups cauliflower rice
- 4 slices bacon, chopped
- 1 small onion, diced
- 1 bell pepper, diced
- 2 cloves garlic, minced
- Salt and pepper to taste
- 2 tbsp olive oil
- 4 eggs (optional, for topping)

Prep Time: 10 mins

Cooking Time: 20 mins

Total Time: 30 mins

Servings: 2

Nutrition Facts (per serving, without eggs)

- Calories: 265
- Fat: 21g
- Saturated Fat: 5g
- Cholesterol: 24mg
- Sodium: 307mg

- Carbohydrate: 12g

- Fiber: 3g

- Protein: 7g

Directions

1. Heat a large skillet over medium heat. Add bacon and cook until crispy. Remove bacon and set aside, leaving the fat in the skillet.

2. Add olive oil, onion, bell pepper, and garlic to the skillet. Sauté until softened.

3. Stir in cauliflower rice, salt, and pepper. Cook until the cauliflower is tender, about 5-7 minutes.

4. Return the bacon to the skillet, mixing well.

5. If desired, make four wells in the hash and crack an egg into each. Cover and cook until the eggs are set to your liking.

6. Serve hot, with additional seasoning as needed.

Spinach and Mushroom Frittata

Ingredients:

- 6 eggs

- 1 cup fresh spinach, chopped

- 1 cup mushrooms, sliced

- ½ cup feta cheese, crumbled

- ¼ cup milk

- 2 tbsp olive oil

- Salt and pepper to taste

Prep Time: 5 mins

Cooking Time: 25 mins

Total Time: 30 mins

Servings: 4

Nutrition Facts (per serving):

- Calories: 220
- Fat: 17g
- Saturated Fat: 6g
- Cholesterol: 284mg
- Sodium: 410mg
- Carbohydrate: 4g
- Fiber: 1g
- Protein: 14g

Directions

1. Preheat the oven to 375°F (190°C).
2. In a mixing bowl, whisk together eggs, milk, salt, and pepper.
3. Heat olive oil in an oven-safe skillet over medium heat. Add mushrooms and sauté until they begin to brown.
4. Add spinach and cook until wilted.
5. Pour the egg mixture over the vegetables in the skillet. Sprinkle feta cheese on top.
6. Cook without stirring for about 5 minutes, until the edges begin to set.
7. Transfer the skillet to the oven and bake for 15-20 minutes, or until the frittata is set and lightly golden on top.
8. Serve warm, cut into wedges.

Keto Blueberry Muffins

Ingredients:

- 1 ½ cups almond flour
- ½ cup erythritol (or sweetener of choice)
- 2 tsp baking powder

- ⅓ cup unsalted butter, melted
- ⅓ cup unsweetened almond milk
- 3 large eggs
- 1 tsp vanilla extract
- ½ cup blueberries

Prep Time: 10 mins

Cooking Time: 25 mins

Total Time: 35 mins

Servings: 12 muffins

Nutrition Facts (per muffin)

- Calories: 145
- Fat: 13g
- Saturated Fat: 4g
- Cholesterol: 56mg
- Sodium: 113mg
- Carbohydrate: 4g
- Fiber: 2g
- Protein: 4g

Directions:

1. Preheat the oven to 350°F (175°C). Line a muffin tin with paper liners or grease with butter.
2. In a large bowl, mix almond flour, erythritol, and baking powder.
3. In another bowl, whisk together melted butter, almond milk, eggs, and vanilla extract.
4. Combine the wet and dry ingredients until just mixed. Gently fold in the blueberries.
5. Divide the batter evenly among the muffin cups.

6. Bake for 20-25 minutes, or until a toothpick inserted into the centre of a muffin comes out clean.

7. Let cool before serving.

Smoked Salmon Avocado Boats

Ingredients:

- 2 avocados, halved and pitted
- 4 oz smoked salmon, thinly sliced
- 1 tbsp capers
- 1 tbsp red onion, finely chopped
- 1 tbsp lemon juice
- Salt and pepper to taste
- Fresh dill for garnish

Prep Time: 10 mins

Cooking Time: 0 mins

Total Time: 10 mins

Servings: 4 halves

Nutrition Facts (per half):

- Calories: 230
- Fat: 19g
- Saturated Fat: 3g
- Cholesterol: 11mg
- Sodium: 297mg
- Carbohydrate: 9g
- Fiber: 7g
- Protein: 9g

Directions:

1. Use a spoon to slightly hollow out the center of each avocado half, leaving enough flesh to maintain its structure.

2. Drizzle lemon juice over the avocado halves to prevent browning.

3. Arrange smoked salmon slices inside each avocado half.

4. Sprinkle capers and red onion over the top. Season with salt and pepper.

5. Garnish with fresh dill before serving. Enjoy as a refreshing and nutritious breakfast or brunch option.

Lemon Herb Grilled Chicken

Ingredients:

- 4 boneless, skinless chicken breasts
- 2 tablespoons olive oil
- Juice and zest of 1 lemon
- 2 cloves garlic, minced
- 1 teaspoon dried oregano
- 1 teaspoon dried thyme
- Salt and pepper to taste

Prep Time: 15 mins (plus marinating time)

Cooking Time: 20 mins

Total Time: 35 mins (plus marinating time)

Servings: 4

Nutrition Facts (per serving):

- Calories: 220
- Fat: 10g

- Saturated Fat: 1.5g
- Cholesterol: 65mg
- Sodium: 75mg
- Carbohydrate: 2g
- Fiber: 0.5g
- Protein: 29g

Directions:

1. In a bowl, whisk together olive oil, lemon juice and zest, garlic, oregano, thyme, salt, and pepper.

2. Place chicken breasts in a resealable plastic bag or shallow dish. Pour marinade over chicken, ensuring each piece is well-coated. Refrigerate for at least 1 hour, or overnight for best flavor.

3. Preheat grill to medium-high heat. Remove chicken from marinade, discarding any excess marinade.

4. Grill chicken for 10 minutes on each side, or until internal temperature reaches 165°F (74°C).

5. Let chicken rest for 5 minutes before serving. Garnish with additional lemon slices or fresh herbs if desired.

Creamy Garlic Shrimp

Ingredients:

- 1 pound large shrimp, peeled and deveined
- 2 tablespoons butter
- 5 cloves garlic, minced
- 1 cup heavy cream
- 1/2 teaspoon paprika
- Salt and pepper to taste
- 2 tablespoons fresh parsley, chopped
- 1 tablespoon lemon juice

Prep Time: 10 mins

Cooking Time: 10 mins

Total Time: 20 mins

Servings: 4

Nutrition Facts (per serving):

- Calories: 310

- Fat: 24g

- Saturated Fat: 15g

- Cholesterol: 265mg

- Sodium: 880mg

- Carbohydrate: 3g

- Fiber: 0g

- Protein: 20g

Directions:

1. Melt butter in a large skillet over medium heat. Add garlic and sauté until fragrant, about 1 minute.

2. Add shrimp to the skillet, seasoning with paprika, salt, and pepper. Cook until shrimp turn pink and opaque, about 2-3 minutes per side.

3. Pour in heavy cream and bring to a simmer. Let cook for an additional 2-3 minutes, or until the sauce thickens slightly.

4. Stir in lemon juice and parsley. Adjust seasoning if necessary.

5. Serve immediately, garnished with more parsley if desired.

Eggplant Lasagna

Ingredients:

- 2 large eggplants, sliced lengthwise 1/4 inch thick

- 2 cups ricotta cheese

- 1 egg
- 1/2 cup grated Parmesan cheese
- 2 cups spinach, chopped
- 2 cups marinara sauce, low carb
- 2 cups shredded mozzarella cheese
- Salt and pepper to taste
- Olive oil for brushing

Prep Time: 20 mins

Cooking Time: 45 mins

Total Time: 65 mins

Servings: 6

Nutrition Facts (per serving):

- Calories: 350
- Fat: 22g
- Saturated Fat: 12g
- Cholesterol: 90mg
- Sodium: 700mg
- Carbohydrate: 15g
- Fiber: 5g
- Protein: 25g

Directions

1. Preheat oven to 375°F (190°C). Brush eggplant slices with olive oil and season with salt and pepper. Arrange on a baking sheet and bake for 15 minutes, until slightly tender.

2. In a bowl, mix ricotta cheese, egg, Parmesan cheese, and spinach. Season with salt and pepper.

3. Spread a thin layer of marinara sauce on the bottom of a baking dish. Layer eggplant slices, ricotta mixture,

mozzarella cheese, and marinara sauce. Repeat layers until all ingredients are used, finishing with a layer of cheese.

4. Bake in preheated oven for 30 minutes, or until bubbly and golden brown. Let cool for 10 minutes before serving.

Cauliflower Steak with Herb Sauce

Ingredients:

- 2 large heads cauliflower
- 3 tablespoons olive oil
- Salt and pepper to taste

For the Herb Sauce:

- 1/2 cup fresh parsley, chopped
- 1/4 cup fresh cilantro, chopped
- 2 tablespoons fresh chives, chopped
- 1 garlic clove, minced
- Juice of 1 lemon
- 1/4 cup olive oil
- Salt and pepper to taste

Prep Time: 15 mins

Cooking Time: 25 mins

Total Time: 40 mins

Servings: 4

Nutrition Facts (per serving):

- Calories: 250
- Fat: 21g
- Saturated Fat: 3g
- Cholesterol: 0mg
- Sodium: 75mg

- Carbohydrate: 15g

- Fiber: 6g

- Protein: 5g

Directions:

1. Preheat oven to 400°F (200°C). Slice cauliflower heads into 1-inch thick steaks, keeping the stem intact to hold the steaks together.

2. Brush both sides of cauliflower steaks with olive oil and season with salt and pepper. Place on a baking sheet.

3. Roast in the oven for 25 minutes, flipping halfway through, until tender and golden.

4. While the cauliflower cooks, prepare the herb sauce by combining parsley, cilantro, chives, garlic, lemon juice, olive oil, salt, and pepper in a bowl.

5. Serve cauliflower steaks drizzled with the herb sauce.

Zucchini Noodles with Pesto

Ingredients:

- 4 medium zucchinis, spiralized

- 1 cup basil leaves

- 1/3 cup grated Parmesan cheese

- 1/4 cup pine nuts

- 2 cloves garlic

- 1/2 cup olive oil

- Salt and pepper to taste

Prep Time: 15 mins

Cooking Time: 5 mins

Total Time: 20 mins

Servings: 4

Nutrition Facts (per serving):

- Calories: 290
- Fat: 27g
- Saturated Fat: 4g
- Cholesterol: 5mg
- Sodium: 200mg
- Carbohydrate: 8g
- Fiber: 2g
- Protein: 6g

Directions:

1. To make the pesto, combine basil leaves, Parmesan cheese, pine nuts, and garlic in a food processor. Pulse until coarsely chopped.

2. With the processor running, slowly add olive oil until the pesto reaches a smooth consistency. Season with salt and pepper.

3. In a large skillet over medium heat, cook spiralized zucchini noodles for 2-3 minutes, until just tender.

4. Remove from heat and toss with the prepared pesto sauce.

5. Serve immediately, garnished with additional Parmesan cheese if desired.

LUNCH RECIPES

Chicken Caesar Lettuce Wraps

Ingredients:

- 2 cups cooked chicken breast, shredded
- 6 large romaine lettuce leaves
- 1/2 cup Caesar dressing, low carb
- 1/4 cup Parmesan cheese, shaved
- 1/4 cup croutons, low carb (optional)
- Black pepper to taste

Prep Time: 10 mins

Cooking Time: 0 mins

Total Time: 10 mins

Servings: 2

Nutrition Facts (per serving):

- Calories: 365
- Fat: 25g
- Saturated Fat: 6g
- Cholesterol: 105mg
- Sodium: 690mg
- Carbohydrate: 6g
- Protein: 30g
- Fiber: 2g

Directions:

1. Lay out the romaine lettuce leaves on a clean surface.
2. In a bowl, mix the shredded chicken with Caesar dressing until well coated.
3. Divide the chicken mixture evenly among the lettuce leaves.

4. Top each wrap with Parmesan cheese, croutons (if using), and a sprinkle of black pepper.

5. Serve immediately, rolling the lettuce around the filling to eat.

Avocado Tuna Salad

Ingredients:

- 2 cans (5 oz each) tuna in water, drained

- 1 ripe avocado, mashed

- 1/4 cup red onion, finely chopped

- 1/4 cup celery, finely chopped

- 2 tablespoons mayonnaise, low carb

- 1 tablespoon lemon juice

- Salt and pepper to taste

- Lettuce leaves for serving

Prep Time: 15 mins

Cooking Time: 0 mins

Total Time: 15 mins

Servings: 4

Nutrition Facts (per serving):

- Calories: 220

- Fat: 14g

- Saturated Fat: 2.5g

- Cholesterol: 30mg

- Sodium: 390mg

- Carbohydrate: 6g

- Protein: 20g

- Fiber: 4g

Directions:

1. In a mixing bowl, combine the mashed avocado, mayonnaise, and lemon juice. Mix until smooth.

2. Add the drained tuna, red onion, and celery to the avocado mixture. Stir to combine thoroughly.

3. Season with salt and pepper to taste.

4. Serve the tuna salad on lettuce leaves or as a filling for low-carb sandwiches.

Beef and Broccoli Stir-Fry

Ingredients:

- 1 lb beef sirloin, thinly sliced
- 2 cups broccoli florets
- 2 tablespoons olive oil
- 1/4 cup soy sauce, low sodium
- 1 tablespoon ginger, minced
- 2 cloves garlic, minced
- 1 tablespoon sesame oil
- 1 teaspoon erythritol (or sweetener of choice)
- 1/2 teaspoon xanthan gum (for thickening)
- Sesame seeds for garnish

Prep Time: 15 mins

Cooking Time: 10 mins

Total Time: 25 mins

Servings: 4

Nutrition Facts (per serving):

- Calories: 280
- Fat: 18g

- Saturated Fat: 4g

- Cholesterol: 70mg

- Sodium: 630mg

- Carbohydrate: 6g

- Protein: 24g

- Fiber: 2g

Directions:

1. Heat olive oil in a large skillet or wok over medium-high heat. Add the beef and stir-fry until browned and cooked through, about 3-4 minutes. Remove beef and set aside.

2. In the same skillet, add broccoli, ginger, and garlic. Stir-fry for 2-3 minutes, or until the broccoli is tender-crisp.

3. Return the beef to the skillet. Add soy sauce, sesame oil, erythritol, and xanthan gum. Stir well to combine and cook until the sauce thickens, about 2 minutes.

4. Garnish with sesame seeds before serving.

Spinach and Goat Cheese Stuffed Chicken

Ingredients:

- 4 boneless, skinless chicken breasts

- 1 cup spinach, cooked and squeezed dry

- 1/2 cup goat cheese, crumbled

- 2 tablespoons olive oil

- Salt and pepper to taste

- 1 teaspoon garlic powder

- 1/2 teaspoon paprika

Prep Time: 20 mins

Cooking Time: 25 mins

Total Time: 45 mins

Servings: 4

Nutrition Facts (per serving):

- Calories: 310
- Fat: 16g
- Saturated Fat: 6g
- Cholesterol: 110mg
- Sodium: 320mg
- Carbohydrate: 2g
- Protein: 38g
- Fiber: 0.5g

Directions:

1. Preheat oven to 375°F (190°C).
2. Cut a pocket into each chicken breast. Stuff each with equal amounts of spinach and goat cheese. Secure with toothpicks if necessary.
3. Season the outside of the chicken with salt, pepper, garlic powder, and paprika.
4. Heat olive oil in an oven-safe skillet over medium-high heat. Sear chicken on both sides until golden, about 3 minutes per side.
5. Transfer skillet to the oven and bake for 20 minutes, or until chicken is cooked through.
6. Remove toothpicks and serve hot.

Shrimp and Avocado Salad

Ingredients:

- 1 lb shrimp, peeled and deveined
- 2 ripe avocados, diced
- 1/4 cup red onion, finely chopped
- 1/2 cup cucumber, diced

- 1/4 cup cilantro, chopped, Juice of 2 limes
- 2 tablespoons olive oil
- Salt and pepper to taste

Prep Time: 15 mins

Cooking Time: 5 mins

Total Time: 20 mins

Servings: 4

Nutrition Facts (per serving):

- Calories: 295
- Fat: 20g
- Saturated Fat: 3g
- Cholesterol: 143mg
- Sodium: 117mg
- Carbohydrate: 10g
- Protein: 20g
- Fiber: 7g

Directions:

1. Cook shrimp in boiling water until pink and opaque, about 2-3 minutes. Drain and let cool.
2. In a large bowl, combine cooled shrimp, diced avocados, red onion, cucumber, and cilantro.
3. In a small bowl, whisk together lime juice, olive oil, salt, and pepper. Pour over the shrimp and avocado mixture.
4. Gently toss to combine. Serve chilled or at room temperature.

Grilled Salmon with Asparagus

Ingredients:

- 4 salmon fillets (6 oz each)

- 1 lb asparagus, ends trimmed
- 2 tablespoons olive oil
- Salt and pepper to taste
- 1 lemon, sliced
- 2 tablespoons fresh dill, chopped

Prep Time: 10 mins

Cooking Time: 15 mins

Total Time: 25 mins

Servings: 4

Nutrition Facts (per serving):

- Calories: 345
- Fat: 20g
- Saturated Fat: 3g
- Cholesterol: 94mg
- Sodium: 75mg
- Carbohydrate: 5g
- Protein: 34g
- Fiber: 2g

Directions:

1. Preheat grill to medium-high heat. Brush salmon and asparagus with olive oil and season with salt and pepper.

2. Place salmon, skin-side down, on the grill. Arrange asparagus around salmon. Grill salmon for 6-8 minutes per side or until cooked through. Grill asparagus for about 5 minutes, turning occasionally, until tender and charred.

3. Serve salmon and asparagus garnished with lemon slices and sprinkled with fresh dill.

Keto Cobb Salad

Ingredients:

- 6 cups mixed greens
- 1 cup cherry tomatoes, halved
- 1 avocado, diced
- 4 hard-boiled eggs, quartered
- 6 slices bacon, cooked and crumbled
- 1 cup cooked chicken breast, diced
- 1/2 cup blue cheese, crumbled
- 1/4 cup red onion, thinly sliced

For the dressing:

- 1/3 cup olive oil
- 3 tablespoons red wine vinegar
- 1 teaspoon Dijon mustard
- Salt and pepper to taste

Prep Time: 20 mins

Cooking Time: 0 mins

Total Time: 20 mins

Servings: 4

Nutrition Facts (per serving):

- Calories: 540
- Fat: 42g
- Saturated Fat: 12g
- Cholesterol: 275mg
- Sodium: 710mg
- Carbohydrate: 12g
- Protein: 33g
- Fiber: 7g

Directions:

1. Arrange mixed greens in a large serving bowl. Top with rows of cherry tomatoes, avocado, hard-boiled eggs, bacon, chicken, blue cheese, and red onion.

2. In a small bowl, whisk together olive oil, red wine vinegar, Dijon mustard, salt, and pepper to make the dressing.

3. Drizzle dressing over the salad just before serving. Toss to combine or serve as is for a classic Cobb presentation.

Zucchini Boat Pizzas

Ingredients:

- 4 medium zucchinis, halved lengthwise
- 1 cup marinara sauce, low carb
- 1 cup mozzarella cheese, shredded
- 1/2 cup mini pepperoni slices
- 1 tablespoon olive oil
- Salt and pepper to taste
- Fresh basil for garnish

Prep Time: 10 mins

Cooking Time: 20 mins

Total Time: 30 mins

Servings: 4

Nutrition Facts (per serving):

- Calories: 250
- Fat: 18g
- Saturated Fat: 6g
- Cholesterol: 35mg
- Sodium: 540mg
- Carbohydrate: 8g

- Protein: 15g
- Fiber: 2g

Directions:

1. Preheat oven to 400°F (200°C). Scoop out the center of each zucchini half to create a "boat."
2. Brush the inside of each zucchini boat with olive oil and season with salt and pepper. Place on a baking sheet.
3. Spoon marinara sauce into each zucchini boat. Top with mozzarella cheese and mini pepperoni slices.
4. Bake in the preheated oven for 20 minutes, or until zucchini is tender and cheese is melted and bubbly.
5. Garnish with fresh basil before serving.

Cauliflower Fried Rice

Ingredients:

- 1 head cauliflower, riced
- 2 tablespoons sesame oil
- 1 small onion, diced
- 1 cup mixed vegetables (carrots, peas, corn), thawed
- 2 cloves garlic, minced
- 2 eggs, lightly beaten
- 3 tablespoons soy sauce, low sodium
- Salt and pepper to taste
- 2 green onions, sliced

Prep Time: 15 mins

Cooking Time: 10 mins

Total Time: 25 mins

Servings: 4

Nutrition Facts (per serving):

- Calories: 175
- Fat: 11g
- Saturated Fat: 2g
- Cholesterol: 93mg
- Sodium: 510mg
- Carbohydrate: 13g
- Protein: 8g
- Fiber: 4g

Directions:

1. Heat sesame oil in a large skillet over medium heat. Add onion and mixed vegetables, cooking until softened, about 5 minutes.

2. Add garlic and riced cauliflower, stirring to combine. Cook for an additional 5 minutes, or until cauliflower is tender.

3. Push cauliflower mixture to the side of the skillet. Add eggs to the other side and scramble until set.

4. Stir scrambled eggs into the cauliflower mixture. Add soy sauce, salt, and pepper, mixing well.

5. Garnish with green onions before serving.

Turkey Lettuce Wraps

Ingredients:

- 1 lb ground turkey,1 tablespoon olive oil
- 1 bell pepper, diced
- 1 onion, diced, 2 cloves garlic, minced
- 1 tablespoon ginger, minced
- 1/4 cup hoisin sauce, low carb
- 1 tablespoon soy sauce, low sodium
- 1 tablespoon rice vinegar

- 1 teaspoon sesame oil
- 1 head iceberg lettuce, leaves separated
- Fresh cilantro for garnish

Prep Time: 15 mins

Cooking Time: 10 mins

Total Time: 25 mins

Servings: 4

Nutrition Facts (per serving):

- Calories: 235
- Fat: 13g
- Saturated Fat: 3g
- Cholesterol: 62mg
- Sodium: 420mg
- Carbohydrate: 8g
- Protein: 23g
- Fiber: 2g

Directions:

1. Heat olive oil in a skillet over medium heat. Add ground turkey, cooking until browned and crumbled.

2. Add bell pepper, onion, garlic, and ginger to the skillet. Cook until vegetables are softened, about 5 minutes.

3. Stir in hoisin sauce, soy sauce, rice vinegar, and sesame oil. Cook for an additional 2 minutes, allowing flavors to meld.

4. Spoon turkey mixture into lettuce leaves. Garnish with fresh cilantro before serving.

Stuffed Bell Peppers

Ingredients:

- 4 large bell peppers, tops removed and seeded

- 1 lb ground beef
- 1 tablespoon olive oil
- 1/2 cup onion, chopped
- 2 cloves garlic, minced
- 1 cup cauliflower rice
- 1 cup diced tomatoes, drained
- 1 teaspoon cumin
- 1 teaspoon paprika
- Salt and pepper to taste
- 1/2 cup shredded cheddar cheese

Prep Time: 15 mins

Cooking Time: 30 mins

Total Time: 45 mins

Servings: 4

Nutrition Facts (per serving):

- Calories: 350
- Fat: 22g
- Saturated Fat: 9g
- Cholesterol: 80mg
- Sodium: 320mg
- Carbohydrate: 15g
- Protein: 25g
- Fiber: 4g

Directions:

1. Preheat oven to 375°F (190°C). Place bell peppers in a baking dish, cut-side up.

2. Heat olive oil in a skillet over medium heat. Add onion and garlic, sautéing until softened.

3. Add ground beef, breaking it apart with a spoon, and cook until browned.

4. Stir in cauliflower rice, diced tomatoes, cumin, paprika, salt, and pepper. Cook for 5 minutes, until flavors meld.

5. Spoon the beef mixture into each bell pepper. Top with shredded cheddar cheese.

6. Bake in the preheated oven for 25-30 minutes, or until peppers are tender and cheese is melted.

7. Serve hot, garnished with fresh herbs if desired.

Creamy Spinach Stuffed Mushrooms

Ingredients:

- 12 large mushrooms, stems removed
- 1 tablespoon olive oil
- 2 cups spinach, chopped
- 1/2 cup cream cheese, softened
- 1/4 cup grated Parmesan cheese
- 2 cloves garlic, minced
- Salt and pepper to taste
- 1/4 cup mozzarella cheese, shredded

Prep Time: 20 mins

Cooking Time: 20 mins

Total Time: 40 mins

Servings: 4 (3 mushrooms each)

Nutrition Facts (per serving):

- Calories: 220
- Fat: 18g

- Saturated Fat: 9g
- Cholesterol: 45mg
- Sodium: 380mg
- Carbohydrate: 6g
- Protein: 9g
- Fiber: 1g

Directions:

1. Preheat oven to 350°F (175°C). Arrange mushroom caps on a baking sheet.
2. Heat olive oil in a skillet over medium heat. Add spinach and garlic, cooking until spinach is wilted.
3. In a bowl, mix together the cooked spinach, cream cheese, Parmesan cheese, salt, and pepper.
4. Fill each mushroom cap with the spinach mixture. Top with shredded mozzarella cheese.
5. Bake in the preheated oven for 20 minutes, or until mushrooms are tender and cheese is golden.
6. Serve warm as a delicious and nutritious appetizer or side dish.

Lemon Garlic Butter Shrimp Skewers

Ingredients:

- 1 lb large shrimp, peeled and deveined
- 2 tablespoons olive oil
- Juice and zest of 1 lemon
- 3 cloves garlic, minced
- 1 tablespoon butter, melted
- Salt and pepper to taste
- Fresh parsley, chopped for garnish

Prep Time: 15 mins (plus marinating time)

Cooking Time: 6 mins

Total Time: 21 mins

Servings: 4

Nutrition Facts (per serving):

- Calories: 210
- Fat: 12g
- Saturated Fat: 3g
- Cholesterol: 145mg
- Sodium: 880mg
- Carbohydrate: 2g
- Protein: 23g
- Fiber: 0g

Directions:

1. In a bowl, whisk together olive oil, lemon juice and zest, garlic, melted butter, salt, and pepper.

2. Add shrimp to the marinade, ensuring they are well coated. Cover and refrigerate for at least 30 minutes.

3. Preheat grill to medium-high heat. Thread shrimp onto skewers.

4. Grill shrimp skewers for 2-3 minutes on each side, or until shrimp are pink and opaque.

5. Garnish with fresh parsley before serving. Serve with a side of low-carb vegetables or salad for a complete meal.

Asian Chicken Salad

Ingredients:

- 2 cups cooked chicken breast, shredded
- 4 cups mixed salad greens
- 1 cup red cabbage, shredded

- 1/2 cup cucumber, sliced
- 1/4 cup almonds, sliced
- 2 green onions, sliced

For the dressing:

- 2 tablespoons soy sauce, low sodium
- 1 tablespoon sesame oil
- 1 tablespoon rice vinegar
- 1 teaspoon erythritol (or sweetener of choice)
- 1 teaspoon ginger, grated
- 1 clove garlic, minced

Prep Time: 20 mins

Cooking Time: 0 mins

Total Time: 20 mins

Servings: 4

Nutrition Facts (per serving):

- Calories: 225
- Fat: 12g
- Saturated Fat: 2g
- Cholesterol: 60mg
- Sodium: 320mg
- Carbohydrate: 6g
- Protein: 24g
- Fiber: 3g

Directions:

1. In a large salad bowl, combine shredded chicken, mixed salad greens, red cabbage, cucumber, almonds, and green onions.

2. In a small bowl, whisk together soy sauce, sesame oil, rice vinegar, erythritol, ginger, and garlic to make the dressing.

3. Drizzle the dressing over the salad and toss to combine.

4. Serve immediately, offering a refreshing and protein-packed lunch option.

Spicy Beef Lettuce Wraps

Ingredients:

- 1 lb ground beef

- 1 tablespoon olive oil

- 1 onion, diced

- 2 cloves garlic, minced

- 1 tablespoon chili powder

- 1 teaspoon cumin

- Salt and pepper to taste

- 1/2 cup tomato sauce, low carb

- 1/4 cup water

- 1 head iceberg lettuce, leaves separated

- Fresh cilantro, chopped for garnish

- Lime wedges for serving

Prep Time: 10 mins

Cooking Time: 15 mins

Total Time: 25 mins

Servings: 4

Nutrition Facts (per serving):

- Calories: 290

- Fat: 20g

- Saturated Fat: 7g

- Cholesterol: 80mg

- Sodium: 320mg

- Carbohydrate: 6g

- Protein: 23g

- Fiber: 2g

Directions:

1. Heat olive oil in a skillet over medium heat. Add onion and garlic, cooking until softened.

2. Add ground beef to the skillet, breaking it apart with a spoon. Cook until browned.

3. Stir in chili powder, cumin, salt, pepper, tomato sauce, and water. Simmer for 10 minutes, or until the sauce has thickened.

4. Spoon the beef mixture into lettuce leaves. Garnish with fresh cilantro.

5. Serve with lime wedges on the side for a zesty and satisfying lunch.

Mediterranean Chicken Skillet

Ingredients:

- 4 boneless, skinless chicken thighs

- 2 tablespoons olive oil

- 1 cup cherry tomatoes, halved

- 1/2 cup Kalamata olives, pitted

- 1/4 cup feta cheese, crumbled

- 2 cloves garlic, minced

- 1 teaspoon dried oregano

- Salt and pepper to taste

- Fresh basil for garnish

- Lemon wedges for serving

Prep Time: 10 mins

Cooking Time: 20 mins

Total Time: 30 mins

Servings: 4

Nutrition Facts (per serving):

- Calories: 300
- Fat: 20g
- Saturated Fat: 5g
- Cholesterol: 110mg
- Sodium: 480mg
- Carbohydrate: 4g
- Protein: 25g
- Fiber: 1g

Directions:

1. Heat olive oil in a large skillet over medium-high heat. Season chicken thighs with salt, pepper, and oregano. Add to the skillet and cook until browned on both sides and cooked through, about 6-8 minutes per side.

2. Add garlic to the skillet and cook until fragrant, about 1 minute. Add cherry tomatoes and olives, cooking until tomatoes are just starting to soften, about 3-4 minutes.

3. Sprinkle feta cheese over the chicken and vegetables. Cover and cook for an additional 2 minutes, or until cheese is slightly melted.

4. Garnish with fresh basil and serve with lemon wedges on the side.

Cauliflower Mac and Cheese

Ingredients:

- 1 large head cauliflower, cut into small florets

- 2 tablespoons butter

- 2 cloves garlic, minced

- 1 cup heavy cream

- 1 1/2 cups sharp cheddar cheese, shredded

- 1/2 cup grated Parmesan cheese

- Salt and pepper to taste

- 1/4 teaspoon paprika

- Fresh parsley, chopped for garnish

Prep Time: 10 mins

Cooking Time: 20 mins

Total Time: 30 mins

Servings: 4

Nutrition Facts (per serving):

- Calories: 450

- Fat: 38g

- Saturated Fat: 24g

- Cholesterol: 120mg

- Sodium: 550mg

- Carbohydrate: 10g

- Protein: 20g

- Fiber: 3g

Directions:

1. Preheat oven to 375°F (190°C). Steam cauliflower florets until tender, about 5-7 minutes. Drain well.

2. In a saucepan, melt butter over medium heat. Add garlic and cook until fragrant, about 1 minute. Stir in heavy cream and bring to a simmer.

3. Reduce heat to low and gradually add cheddar and Parmesan cheeses, stirring until melted and smooth. Season with salt, pepper, and paprika.

4. Add the steamed cauliflower to the cheese sauce, stirring to coat. Transfer to a baking dish.

5. Bake in the preheated oven for 15 minutes, or until bubbly and golden on top.

6. Garnish with fresh parsley before serving.

Spicy Tofu Stir-Fry

Ingredients:

- 1 block (14 oz) firm tofu, pressed and cubed
- 2 tablespoons soy sauce, low sodium
- 1 tablespoon sesame oil
- 1 tablespoon Sriracha or chili sauce
- 2 cups mixed vegetables (bell peppers, broccoli, snap peas)
- 2 cloves garlic, minced
- 1 teaspoon ginger, grated
- 2 green onions, sliced
- Sesame seeds for garnish

Prep Time: 15 mins

Cooking Time: 10 mins

Total Time: 25 mins

Servings: 4

Nutrition Facts (per serving):

- Calories: 180
- Fat: 10g
- Saturated Fat: 1.5g
- Cholesterol: 0mg

- Sodium: 320mg
- Carbohydrate: 10g
- Protein: 12g
- Fiber: 3g

Directions:

1. In a bowl, mix soy sauce, sesame oil, and Sriracha. Add tofu cubes and gently toss to coat. Let marinate for 10 minutes.

2. Heat a large skillet or wok over medium-high heat. Add tofu and cook until all sides are golden brown, about 5-7 minutes. Remove tofu and set aside.

3. In the same skillet, add a bit more sesame oil if needed. Sauté garlic and ginger until fragrant. Add mixed vegetables and stir-fry until just tender.

4. Return tofu to the skillet. Add green onions and toss everything together. Cook for an additional 2 minutes.

5. Serve hot, garnished with sesame seeds.

Turkey and Avocado Club Salad

Ingredients:

- 2 cups cooked turkey breast, chopped
- 1 large avocado, diced
- 1/2 cup cherry tomatoes, halved
- 1/4 cup cooked bacon, crumbled
- 4 cups mixed salad greens

For the dressing:

- 2 tablespoons mayonnaise, low carb
- 1 tablespoon Dijon mustard
- 1 tablespoon apple cider vinegar
- Salt and pepper to taste

Prep Time: 15 mins

Cooking Time: 0 mins

Total Time: 15 mins

Servings: 4

Nutrition Facts (per serving):

- Calories: 290
- Fat: 18g
- Saturated Fat: 3g
- Cholesterol: 70mg
- Sodium: 320mg
- Carbohydrate: 8g
- Protein: 25g
- Fiber: 4g

Directions:

1. In a large salad bowl, combine turkey, avocado, cherry tomatoes, bacon, and mixed salad greens.
2. In a small bowl, whisk together mayonnaise, Dijon mustard, apple cider vinegar, salt, and pepper to create the dressing.
3. Drizzle the dressing over the salad and toss to combine.
4. Serve immediately, offering a refreshing and satisfying meal.

Roasted Vegetable Quiche

Ingredients:

- 1 cup broccoli florets
- 1 red bell pepper, diced
- 1 zucchini, sliced
- 2 tablespoons olive oil
- Salt and pepper to taste
- 6 large eggs

- 1/2 cup heavy cream
- 1 cup shredded Swiss cheese
- 1 teaspoon dried thyme

Prep Time: 20 mins

Cooking Time: 35 mins

Total Time: 55 mins

Servings: 6

Nutrition Facts (per serving):

- Calories: 280
- Fat: 22g
- Saturated Fat: 10g
- Cholesterol: 215mg
- Sodium: 180mg
- Carbohydrate: 5g
- Protein: 16g
- Fiber: 1g

Directions:

1. Preheat oven to 400°F (200°C). Toss broccoli, bell pepper, and zucchini with olive oil, salt, and pepper. Spread on a baking sheet and roast for 15 minutes, until vegetables are tender. Reduce oven temperature to 375°F (190°C).

2. In a large bowl, whisk together eggs, heavy cream, Swiss cheese, thyme, and additional salt and pepper.

3. Spread the roasted vegetables evenly in a greased 9-inch pie dish. Pour the egg mixture over the vegetables.

4. Bake in the preheated oven for 35 minutes, or until the quiche is set and the top is lightly golden.

5. Let cool for a few minutes before slicing and serving.

DINNER RECIPES

Garlic Butter Steak Bites with Zucchini Noodles

Ingredients:

- 1 lb sirloin steak, cut into 1-inch pieces
- 4 medium zucchinis, spiralized
- 4 tablespoons butter, divided
- 3 cloves garlic, minced
- Salt and pepper to taste
- 1 teaspoon Italian seasoning
- 2 tablespoons fresh parsley, chopped
- Juice of 1/2 lemon

Prep Time: 15 mins

Cooking Time: 10 mins

Total Time: 25 mins

Servings: 4

Nutrition Facts (per serving):

- Calories: 325
- Fat: 20g
- Saturated Fat: 9g
- Cholesterol: 105mg
- Sodium: 125mg
- Carbohydrate: 8g
- Protein: 30g
- Fiber: 2g

Directions:

1. Season steak bites with salt, pepper, and Italian seasoning.

2. Heat 2 tablespoons of butter in a large skillet over medium-high heat. Add steak bites and cook until browned on all sides and cooked to your desired doneness, about 3-4 minutes. Remove steak from skillet and set aside.

3. In the same skillet, add the remaining 2 tablespoons of butter and garlic. Sauté for 1 minute until fragrant.

4. Add spiralized zucchini to the skillet, tossing to coat in the garlic butter. Cook for 2-3 minutes until zucchini noodles are tender.

5. Return steak bites to the skillet. Squeeze lemon juice over the top and sprinkle with fresh parsley.

6. Serve immediately, offering a flavourful and satisfying low-carb dinner.

Lemon Herb Roasted Chicken Thighs

Ingredients:

- 8 bone-in, skin-on chicken thighs
- 2 tablespoons olive oil
- Juice and zest of 1 lemon
- 2 cloves garlic, minced
- 1 tablespoon fresh rosemary, chopped
- 1 tablespoon fresh thyme, chopped
- Salt and pepper to taste

Prep Time: 10 mins

Cooking Time: 40 mins

Total Time: 50 mins

Servings: 4

Nutrition Facts (per serving):

- Calories: 475
- Fat: 35g

- Saturated Fat: 9g
- Cholesterol: 195mg
- Sodium: 125mg
- Carbohydrate: 2g
- Protein: 38g
- Fiber: 0.5g

Directions:

1. Preheat oven to 400°F (200°C).
2. In a small bowl, mix together olive oil, lemon juice and zest, garlic, rosemary, thyme, salt, and pepper.
3. Place chicken thighs in a baking dish. Brush each thigh with the lemon herb mixture, ensuring each piece is well-coated.
4. Roast in the preheated oven for 35-40 minutes, or until chicken is golden brown and cooked through (internal temperature of 165°F or 74°C).
5. Serve hot, garnished with additional fresh herbs and lemon slices if desired.

Creamy Tuscan Salmon

Ingredients:

- 4 salmon fillets (6 oz each)
- 2 tablespoons olive oil
- 3 cloves garlic, minced
- 1 cup heavy cream
- 1/2 cup sun-dried tomatoes, chopped
- 2 cups spinach, fresh
- 1/4 cup grated Parmesan cheese
- Salt and pepper to taste
- Fresh basil for garnish

Prep Time: 10 mins

Cooking Time: 20 mins

Total Time: 30 mins

Servings: 4

Nutrition Facts (per serving):

- Calories: 540
- Fat: 40g
- Saturated Fat: 18g
- Cholesterol: 125mg
- Sodium: 320mg
- Carbohydrate: 8g
- Protein: 38g
- Fiber: 1g

Directions:

1. Season salmon fillets with salt and pepper.
2. Heat olive oil in a large skillet over medium-high heat. Add salmon, skin-side up, and cook until golden brown on one side, about 3-4 minutes. Flip and cook for an additional 3 minutes. Remove salmon from skillet and set aside.
3. In the same skillet, add garlic and sauté until fragrant. Stir in heavy cream, sun-dried tomatoes, and Parmesan cheese. Simmer for 5 minutes, until the sauce thickens slightly.
4. Add spinach to the skillet, cooking until wilted. Return salmon to the skillet, spooning the sauce over the fillets.
5. Garnish with fresh basil before serving. Enjoy a luxurious and hearty meal that's still low in carbs.

Eggplant Parmesan Casserole

Ingredients:

- 2 large eggplants, sliced into 1/2-inch rounds

- 2 cups marinara sauce, low carb
- 2 cups shredded mozzarella cheese
- 1/2 cup grated Parmesan cheese
- 1/4 cup fresh basil, chopped
- 2 tablespoons olive oil
- Salt and pepper to taste

Prep Time: 15 mins

Cooking Time: 45 mins

Total Time: 60 mins

Servings: 6

Nutrition Facts (per serving):

- Calories: 290
- Fat: 18g
- Saturated Fat: 8g
- Cholesterol: 40mg
- Sodium: 520mg
- Carbohydrate: 15g
- Protein: 18g
- Fiber: 6g

Directions:

1. Preheat oven to 375°F (190°C). Brush eggplant slices with olive oil and season with salt and pepper. Arrange on baking sheets in a single layer.

2. Bake eggplant slices for 25 minutes, flipping halfway through, until tender and slightly golden.

3. In a baking dish, spread a thin layer of marinara sauce. Layer baked eggplant slices, more sauce, mozzarella, and Parmesan cheese. Repeat layers, finishing with cheese on top.

4. Bake in the preheated oven for 20 minutes, or until the cheese is bubbly and golden.

5. Garnish with fresh basil before serving. This dish offers all the flavours of traditional eggplant Parmesan but in a low-carb, comforting casserole form.

Shrimp and Cauliflower Grits

Ingredients:

- 1 lb large shrimp, peeled and deveined
- 4 cups cauliflower rice
- 1 cup chicken broth, 1/2 cup heavy cream
- 1/2 cup grated cheddar cheese
- 2 tablespoons butter, 2 cloves garlic, minced
- 1 teaspoon paprika
- Salt and pepper to taste
- Green onions, sliced for garnish

Prep Time: 15 mins

Cooking Time: 20 mins

Total Time: 35 mins

Servings: 4

Nutrition Facts (per serving):

- Calories: 330
- Fat: 22g
- Saturated Fat: 13g
- Cholesterol: 245mg
- Sodium: 880mg
- Carbohydrate: 10g
- Protein: 25g
- Fiber: 3g

Directions:

1. In a large skillet, melt butter over medium heat. Add garlic and shrimp. Season with paprika, salt, and pepper. Cook until shrimp are pink and opaque, about 3-4 minutes per side. Remove shrimp from skillet and set aside.

2. In the same skillet, add cauliflower rice and chicken broth. Cook until the cauliflower is tender and most of the liquid has been absorbed, about 5-7 minutes.

3. Stir in heavy cream and cheddar cheese until the cheese is melted and the mixture resembles grits in texture.

4. Serve shrimp over cauliflower grits. Garnish with sliced green onions. This dish provides a comforting, Southern-inspired meal without the high carb count of traditional grits.

Pork Chops with Creamy Mushroom Sauce

Ingredients:

- 4 boneless pork chops
- 2 tablespoons olive oil
- Salt and pepper to taste
- 1 cup mushrooms, sliced
- 2 cloves garlic, minced
- 1/2 cup chicken broth
- 1/2 cup heavy cream
- 1 teaspoon Dijon mustard
- 1 tablespoon fresh thyme, chopped

Prep Time: 10 mins

Cooking Time: 20 mins

Total Time: 30 mins

Servings: 4

Nutrition Facts (per serving):

- Calories: 380
- Fat: 28g
- Saturated Fat: 12g
- Cholesterol: 125mg
- Sodium: 220mg
- Carbohydrate: 3g
- Protein: 29g
- Fiber: 0.5g

Directions:

1. Season pork chops with salt and pepper. Heat olive oil in a large skillet over medium-high heat. Add pork chops and cook until golden brown on both sides and cooked through, about 6-8 minutes per side. Remove from skillet and set aside.

2. In the same skillet, add mushrooms and garlic. Cook until mushrooms are golden and garlic is fragrant, about 3-4 minutes.

3. Pour in chicken broth to deglaze the pan, scraping up any browned bits. Stir in heavy cream, Dijon mustard, and thyme. Simmer until the sauce thickens, about 5 minutes.

4. Return pork chops to the skillet, spooning the sauce over them. Cook for an additional 2-3 minutes, until pork chops are heated through.

5. Serve pork chops with the creamy mushroom sauce spooned over the top.

Spicy Chicken and Avocado Wraps

Ingredients:

- 2 cups cooked chicken breast, shredded
- 1 avocado, diced
- 1/2 cup cherry tomatoes, halved

- 1/4 cup red onion, finely chopped
- 1 jalapeño, seeded and finely chopped
- 2 tablespoons cilantro, chopped
- Juice of 1 lime
- Salt and pepper to taste
- 4 large lettuce leaves (e.g., iceberg or butter lettuce)

Prep Time: 15 mins

Cooking Time: 0 mins

Total Time: 15 mins

Servings: 4

Nutrition Facts (per serving):

- Calories: 220
- Fat: 11g
- Saturated Fat: 2g
- Cholesterol: 60mg
- Sodium: 70mg
- Carbohydrate: 6g
- Protein: 25g
- Fiber: 4g

Directions:

1. In a large bowl, combine shredded chicken, avocado, cherry tomatoes, red onion, jalapeño, and cilantro. Drizzle with lime juice and season with salt and pepper. Toss gently to combine.

2. Place a scoop of the chicken mixture onto the center of each lettuce leaf. Fold the sides of the lettuce over the filling, then roll up to enclose.

3. Serve immediately, offering a refreshing and spicy twist on the traditional wrap.

Balsamic Roasted Brussels Sprouts

Ingredients:

- 1 lb Brussels sprouts, trimmed and halved
- 2 tablespoons olive oil
- Salt and pepper to taste
- 2 tablespoons balsamic vinegar
- 1 tablespoon grated Parmesan cheese

Prep Time: 10 mins

Cooking Time: 25 mins

Total Time: 35 mins

Servings: 4

Nutrition Facts (per serving):

- Calories: 120
- Fat: 7g
- Saturated Fat: 1g
- Cholesterol: 1mg
- Sodium: 75mg
- Carbohydrate: 10g
- Protein: 4g
- Fiber: 4g

Directions:

1. Preheat oven to 400°F (200°C). Toss Brussels sprouts with olive oil, salt, and pepper. Spread on a baking sheet in a single layer.

2. Roast in the preheated oven for 20-25 minutes, stirring halfway through, until Brussels sprouts are tender and caramelized.

3. Drizzle balsamic vinegar over the roasted Brussels sprouts and toss to coat evenly.

4. Sprinkle grated Parmesan cheese over the top before serving. Enjoy a flavourful and nutritious side dish that pairs well with any protein.

Grilled Eggplant with Tomato and Feta

Ingredients:

- 2 large eggplants, sliced into 1/2-inch rounds
- 1/4 cup olive oil
- Salt and pepper to taste
- 2 tomatoes, sliced
- 1/2 cup feta cheese, crumbled
- 2 tablespoons fresh basil, chopped
- Balsamic glaze for drizzling

Prep Time: 10 mins

Cooking Time: 10 mins

Total Time: 20 mins

Servings: 4

Nutrition Facts (per serving):

- Calories: 230
- Fat: 18g
- Saturated Fat: 5g
- Cholesterol: 25mg
- Sodium: 310mg
- Carbohydrate: 14g
- Protein: 6g
- Fiber: 7g

Directions:

1. Preheat grill to medium-high heat. Brush eggplant slices with olive oil and season with salt and pepper.

2. Grill eggplant slices for 3-4 minutes on each side, until tender and grill marks appear.

3. Arrange grilled eggplant on a serving platter. Top each slice with a tomato slice and sprinkle with crumbled feta cheese.

4. Garnish with chopped basil and drizzle with balsamic glaze before serving. This dish offers a delightful combination of flavours and textures, perfect for a light dinner or appetizer.

Lemon Pepper Tilapia

Ingredients:

- 4 tilapia fillets
- 2 tablespoons olive oil
- Juice and zest of 1 lemon
- 1 teaspoon black pepper
- Salt to taste
- 2 tablespoons fresh parsley, chopped

Prep Time: 5 mins

Cooking Time: 10 mins

Total Time: 15 mins

Servings: 4

Nutrition Facts (per serving):

- Calories: 195
- Fat: 10g
- Saturated Fat: 1.5g
- Cholesterol: 85mg
- Sodium: 65mg
- Carbohydrate: 1g

- Protein: 25g
- Fiber: 0.5g

Directions:

1. Preheat a skillet over medium-high heat and add olive oil.

2. Season tilapia fillets with lemon juice, lemon zest, black pepper, and salt.

3. Place tilapia in the skillet and cook for 4-5 minutes on each side, or until the fish flakes easily with a fork.

4. Garnish with fresh parsley before serving. Enjoy a simple, flavourful, and healthy seafood dish that's perfect for a quick and satisfying dinner.

Herb-Crusted Rack of Lamb

Ingredients:

- 1 rack of lamb (about 8 ribs)
- 2 tablespoons olive oil
- 2 cloves garlic, minced
- 2 tablespoons fresh rosemary, chopped
- 2 tablespoons fresh thyme, chopped
- Salt and pepper to taste
- 1/4 cup Dijon mustard
- 1/2 cup almond flour

Prep Time: 15 mins

Cooking Time: 25 mins

Total Time: 40 mins

Servings: 4

Nutrition Facts (per serving):

- Calories: 410
- Fat: 30g

- Saturated Fat: 10g

- Cholesterol: 105mg

- Sodium: 320mg

- Carbohydrate: 4g

- Protein: 32g

- Fiber: 2g

Directions:

1. Preheat oven to 400°F (200°C). Season the rack of lamb with salt and pepper.

2. In a skillet, heat olive oil over medium-high heat. Sear the rack of lamb on all sides until golden brown, about 3-4 minutes per side. Remove from heat.

3. In a bowl, mix together garlic, rosemary, thyme, and almond flour.

4. Brush the rack of lamb with Dijon mustard, then press the herb-almond flour mixture onto the mustard to coat.

5. Place the rack of lamb on a roasting pan and roast in the preheated oven for 20-25 minutes for medium-rare, or until desired doneness.

6. Let rest for 5 minutes before slicing between the ribs and serving. Enjoy this elegant and flavourful dish that's perfect for a special occasion.

Spaghetti Squash Carbonara

Ingredients:

- 1 large spaghetti squash

- 4 slices bacon, chopped

- 1/2 cup onion, chopped

- 2 cloves garlic, minced

- 2 eggs

- 1/2 cup grated Parmesan cheese

- Salt and pepper to taste
- Fresh parsley, chopped for garnish

Prep Time: 10 mins

Cooking Time: 45 mins

Total Time: 55 mins

Servings: 4

Nutrition Facts (per serving):
- Calories: 235
- Fat: 15g
- Saturated Fat: 6g
- Cholesterol: 115mg
- Sodium: 470mg
- Carbohydrate: 15g
- Protein: 12g
- Fiber: 2g

Directions:

1. Preheat oven to 400°F (200°C). Halve the spaghetti squash lengthwise and scoop out the seeds. Place cut-side down on a baking sheet and roast until tender, about 40 minutes.

2. While the squash is roasting, cook bacon in a skillet over medium heat until crispy. Remove bacon and set aside, leaving the fat in the skillet.

3. Add onion and garlic to the skillet and sauté until softened. Remove from heat.

4. In a bowl, whisk together eggs and Parmesan cheese. Season with salt and pepper.

5. Once the spaghetti squash is done, use a fork to scrape the flesh into strands. Add the squash strands to the skillet with the onion and garlic. Toss to combine.

6. Pour the egg and cheese mixture over the squash while it's still hot, quickly tossing to combine and cook the eggs with the residual heat.

7. Serve garnished with crispy bacon, additional Parmesan cheese, and fresh parsley.

Thai Coconut Curry Chicken

Ingredients:

- 1 lb chicken breast, cut into bite-sized pieces
- 2 tablespoons coconut oil
- 1 onion, sliced
- 2 cloves garlic, minced
- 1 tablespoon ginger, minced
- 1 red bell pepper, sliced
- 1 cup broccoli florets
- 1 can (14 oz) coconut milk
- 2 tablespoons red curry paste
- 1 tablespoon fish sauce
- 1 teaspoon erythritol (or sweetener of choice)
- Juice of 1 lime
- Fresh cilantro for garnish

Prep Time: 15 mins

Cooking Time: 20 mins

Total Time: 35 mins

Servings: 4

Nutrition Facts (per serving):

- Calories: 365
- Fat: 22g
- Saturated Fat: 18g

- Cholesterol: 65mg

- Sodium: 320mg

- Carbohydrate: 10g

- Protein: 28g

- Fiber: 2g

Directions:

1. Heat coconut oil in a large skillet over medium heat. Add chicken and cook until browned. Remove chicken and set aside.

2. In the same skillet, add onion, garlic, and ginger. Sauté until onion is translucent.

3. Add red bell pepper and broccoli, cooking until vegetables are just tender.

4. Stir in coconut milk, red curry paste, fish sauce, and erythritol. Bring to a simmer.

5. Return chicken to the skillet. Simmer everything together for 10 minutes, until chicken is cooked through and sauce has thickened.

6. Stir in lime juice. Serve garnished with fresh cilantro. Enjoy a flavourful and comforting dish that brings the taste of Thailand to your table.

Beef and Broccoli Stir-Fry

Ingredients:

- 1 lb beef sirloin, thinly sliced

- 4 cups broccoli florets

- 2 tablespoons vegetable oil

- 2 cloves garlic, minced

For the sauce:

- 1/4 cup soy sauce, low sodium

- 2 tablespoons oyster sauce

- 1 tablespoon sesame oil

- 1 tablespoon erythritol (or sweetener of choice)

- 1 teaspoon ginger, grated

- 1/2 cup beef broth

- 1 teaspoon xanthan gum (for thickening)

Prep Time: 15 mins

Cooking Time: 10 mins

Total Time: 25 mins

Servings: 4

Nutrition Facts (per serving):

- Calories: 280

- Fat: 16g

- Saturated Fat: 3g

- Cholesterol: 70mg

- Sodium: 630mg

- Carbohydrate: 8g

- Protein: 26g

- Fiber: 2g

Directions:

1. In a bowl, whisk together all the sauce ingredients until well combined. Set aside.

2. Heat 1 tablespoon of vegetable oil in a large skillet or wok over high heat. Add beef and stir-fry until browned and cooked through. Remove beef and set aside.

3. In the same skillet, add the remaining tablespoon of oil and garlic. Sauté for 30 seconds, then add broccoli. Stir-fry until the broccoli is bright green and tender-crisp.

4. Return the beef to the skillet. Pour the sauce over the beef and broccoli. Cook, stirring constantly, until the sauce has thickened and coats the beef and broccoli evenly.

5. Serve immediately, offering a classic and satisfying stir-fry dish that's perfect for a low-carb diet.

Lemon Dill Salmon Foil Packets

Ingredients:

- 4 salmon fillets (6 oz each)
- 2 zucchinis, sliced
- 1 lemon, thinly sliced
- 4 tablespoons butter
- 2 tablespoons fresh dill, chopped
- Salt and pepper to taste
- 4 foil sheets, large enough to wrap the salmon and vegetables

Prep Time: 10 mins

Cooking Time: 20 mins

Total Time: 30 mins

Servings: 4

Nutrition Facts (per serving):

- Calories: 345
- Fat: 23g
- Saturated Fat: 9g
- Cholesterol: 110mg
- Sodium: 125mg
- Carbohydrate: 3g
- Protein: 31g
- Fiber: 1g

Directions:

1. Preheat oven to 400°F (200°C) or prepare a grill for medium heat.

2. Place each salmon fillet on a piece of foil. Season with salt and pepper. Top each with equal amounts of zucchini slices, lemon slices, butter, and fresh dill.

3. Fold the foil over the salmon and vegetables, sealing the edges to create a packet.

4. Bake in the preheated oven or grill over medium heat for 15-20 minutes, until salmon is cooked through and vegetables are tender.

5. Carefully open the packets (watch for steam) and serve immediately, enjoying the moist and flavorful salmon with a hint of lemon and dill.

Chicken Alfredo Zucchini Boats

Ingredients:

- 4 medium zucchinis, halved lengthwise
- 2 cups cooked chicken breast, shredded
- 1 cup Alfredo sauce, low carb
- 1/2 cup mozzarella cheese, shredded
- 1/4 cup Parmesan cheese, grated
- 2 tablespoons olive oil
- Salt and pepper to taste
- 1 tablespoon fresh parsley, chopped for garnish

Prep Time: 15 mins

Cooking Time: 25 mins

Total Time: 40 mins

Servings: 4

Nutrition Facts (per serving):

- Calories: 350
- Fat: 25g
- Saturated Fat: 10g
- Cholesterol: 90mg
- Sodium: 580mg
- Carbohydrate: 8g
- Protein: 25g
- Fiber: 2g

Directions:

1. Preheat oven to 375°F (190°C). Scoop out the center of each zucchini half to create a "boat," leaving about 1/4 inch of zucchini along the sides.

2. Brush the zucchini boats with olive oil and season with salt and pepper. Place on a baking sheet and bake for 10 minutes, until slightly tender.

3. In a bowl, mix together the shredded chicken and Alfredo sauce. Spoon the mixture into the zucchini boats.

4. Top each boat with mozzarella and Parmesan cheeses.

5. Bake in the preheated oven for 15 minutes, or until the cheese is melted and bubbly.

6. Garnish with fresh parsley before serving. Enjoy a low-carb twist on the classic chicken Alfredo, perfect for a satisfying dinner.

Stuffed Bell Peppers with Ground Turkey

Ingredients:

- 4 large bell peppers, tops removed and seeded
- 1 lb ground turkey
- 1 tablespoon olive oil
- 1/2 cup onion, chopped

- 2 cloves garlic, minced
- 1 cup cauliflower rice
- 1 can (14 oz) diced tomatoes, drained
- 1 teaspoon cumin, 1 teaspoon smoked paprika
- Salt and pepper to taste
- 1/2 cup shredded cheddar cheese

Prep Time: 20 mins

Cooking Time: 35 mins

Total Time: 55 mins

Servings: 4

Nutrition Facts (per serving):

- Calories: 330
- Fat: 18g
- Saturated Fat: 6g
- Cholesterol: 80mg
- Sodium: 320mg
- Carbohydrate: 15g
- Protein: 28g
- Fiber: 4g

Directions:

1. Preheat oven to 375°F (190°C). Blanch the bell peppers in boiling water for 5 minutes to soften. Drain and set aside.

2. Heat olive oil in a skillet over medium heat. Add onion and garlic, sautéing until translucent.

3. Add ground turkey, breaking it apart with a spoon. Cook until browned.

4. Stir in cauliflower rice, diced tomatoes, cumin, smoked paprika, salt, and pepper. Cook for 5 minutes, until flavors meld.

5. Spoon the turkey mixture into each bell pepper. Place stuffed peppers in a baking dish.

6. Top each pepper with shredded cheddar cheese.

7. Bake in the preheated oven for 25 minutes, or until the peppers are tender and the cheese is melted.

8. Serve hot, offering a hearty and flavourful low-carb meal.

Creamy Garlic Parmesan Shrimp

Ingredients:

- 1 lb large shrimp, peeled and deveined
- 2 tablespoons butter
- 4 cloves garlic, minced
- 1 cup heavy cream
- 1/2 cup Parmesan cheese, grated
- Salt and pepper to taste
- 1 tablespoon fresh parsley, chopped
- 1 teaspoon lemon zest

Prep Time: 10 mins

Cooking Time: 10 mins

Total Time: 20 mins

Servings: 4

Nutrition Facts (per serving):

- Calories: 390
- Fat: 30g
- Saturated Fat: 18g
- Cholesterol: 295mg

- Sodium: 880mg
- Carbohydrate: 3g
- Protein: 28g
- Fiber: 0g

Directions:

1. Melt butter in a large skillet over medium heat. Add garlic and sauté until fragrant, about 1 minute.

2. Add shrimp to the skillet and cook until they turn pink and opaque, about 2-3 minutes per side. Remove shrimp and set aside.

3. Pour heavy cream into the skillet, bringing it to a simmer. Stir in Parmesan cheese until melted and smooth.

4. Return shrimp to the skillet, tossing to coat in the creamy sauce. Season with salt and pepper.

5. Garnish with fresh parsley and lemon zest before serving. Enjoy a luxurious and creamy shrimp dish that's surprisingly easy to make.

Asian Beef Lettuce Wraps

Ingredients:

- 1 lb ground beef, 1 tablespoon sesame oil
- 2 cloves garlic, minced
- 1 tablespoon ginger, minced
- 1/4 cup soy sauce, low sodium
- 1 tablespoon hoisin sauce
- 1 teaspoon chili paste (optional)
- 1 cup mushrooms, finely chopped
- 1/2 cup water chestnuts, diced
- 1/4 cup green onions, sliced
- 8-10 large lettuce leaves (e.g., Bibb or iceberg)

- Sesame seeds for garnish

Prep Time: 15 mins

Cooking Time: 10 mins

Total Time: 25 mins

Servings: 4

Nutrition Facts (per serving):

- Calories: 280

- Fat: 18g

- Saturated Fat: 6g

- Cholesterol: 70mg

- Sodium: 630mg

- Carbohydrate: 8g

- Protein: 22g

- Fiber: 1g

Directions:

1. Heat sesame oil in a large skillet over medium heat. Add garlic and ginger, sautéing until fragrant.

2. Add ground beef to the skillet, breaking it apart with a spoon. Cook until browned.

3. Stir in soy sauce, hoisin sauce, and chili paste. Add mushrooms and water chestnuts, cooking until tender.

4. Remove from heat and stir in green onions.

5. Spoon the beef mixture into lettuce leaves, folding them over to create wraps.

6. Garnish with sesame seeds before serving. Enjoy a flavorful and healthy meal that's perfect for a light dinner or appetizer.

Roasted Cauliflower Steak with Tahini Sauce

Ingredients:

- 2 large heads cauliflower, sliced into 1-inch thick steaks
- 3 tablespoons olive oil
- Salt and pepper to taste, 1/2 cup tahini
- 2 tablespoons lemon juice, 1 clove garlic, minced
- 2-4 tablespoons water (as needed for consistency)
- 2 tablespoons fresh parsley, chopped

Prep Time: 10 mins

Cooking Time: 25 mins

Total Time: 35 mins

Servings: 4

Nutrition Facts (per serving):
- Calories: 310
- Fat: 25g
- Saturated Fat: 3.5g
- Cholesterol: 0mg
- Sodium: 75mg
- Carbohydrate: 18g
- Protein: 8g
- Fiber: 7g

Directions:

1. Preheat oven to 425°F (220°C). Brush cauliflower steaks with olive oil and season with salt and pepper. Place on a baking sheet.

2. Roast in the preheated oven for 20-25 minutes, flipping halfway through, until golden and tender.

3. While the cauliflower is roasting, whisk together tahini, lemon juice, garlic, and water in a bowl until smooth. Adjust consistency with more water if needed.

4. Serve cauliflower steaks drizzled with tahini sauce and garnished with fresh parsley. Enjoy a delicious and nutritious plant-based meal that's full of flavor.

SALAD RECIPES

Avocado Chicken Salad

Ingredients:

- 2 cups cooked chicken breast, shredded
- 1 large avocado, diced, 1/4 cup Greek yogurt, full-fat
- 2 tablespoons lime juice
- 1/4 cup cilantro, chopped
- 1/2 cup cherry tomatoes, halved
- 1/4 cup red onion, finely chopped
- Salt and pepper to taste

Prep Time: 15 mins

Cooking Time: 0 mins

Total Time: 15 mins

Servings: 4

Nutrition Facts (per serving):

- Calories: 250
- Fat: 13g
- Saturated Fat: 3g
- Cholesterol: 60mg
- Sodium: 70mg
- Carbohydrate: 7g
- Protein: 27g
- Fiber: 4g

Directions:

1. In a large bowl, combine the shredded chicken, diced avocado, Greek yogurt, and lime juice. Mix well until the chicken is evenly coated.

2. Add the cilantro, cherry tomatoes, and red onion to the bowl. Season with salt and pepper to taste. Gently toss to combine all the ingredients.

3. Serve immediately or chill in the refrigerator for 30 minutes before serving to allow flavours to meld. Enjoy a creamy and refreshing salad that's perfect for a light lunch or dinner.

Spinach and Goat Cheese Salad with Walnuts

Ingredients:

- 6 cups fresh spinach leaves
- 1/2 cup goat cheese, crumbled
- 1/2 cup walnuts, toasted and chopped
- 1/4 cup red onion, thinly sliced

For the dressing:

- 3 tablespoons olive oil
- 1 tablespoon balsamic vinegar
- 1 teaspoon Dijon mustard
- Salt and pepper to taste

Prep Time: 10 mins

Cooking Time: 0 mins

Total Time: 10 mins

Servings: 4

Nutrition Facts (per serving):

- Calories: 280
- Fat: 24g
- Saturated Fat: 6g
- Cholesterol: 13mg
- Sodium: 180mg
- Carbohydrate: 8g

- Protein: 9g

- Fiber: 3g

Directions:

1. In a large salad bowl, combine the spinach leaves, crumbled goat cheese, toasted walnuts, and red onion.

2. In a small bowl, whisk together the olive oil, balsamic vinegar, Dijon mustard, salt, and pepper to create the dressing.

3. Drizzle the dressing over the salad and toss gently to coat all the ingredients evenly.

4. Serve immediately, offering a sophisticated and nutrient-rich salad that's both satisfying and low in carbs.

Greek Salad with Grilled Chicken

Ingredients:

- 2 cups cooked chicken breast, diced

- 1 cucumber, diced

- 1 cup cherry tomatoes, halved

- 1/2 cup Kalamata olives, pitted

- 1/2 cup feta cheese, crumbled

- 1/4 cup red onion, thinly sliced

For the dressing:

- 3 tablespoons olive oil

- 1 tablespoon red wine vinegar

- 1 teaspoon dried oregano

- Salt and pepper to taste

Prep Time: 20 mins

Cooking Time: 0 mins

Total Time: 20 mins

Servings: 4

Nutrition Facts (per serving):

- Calories: 320
- Fat: 20g
- Saturated Fat: 6g
- Cholesterol: 85mg
- Sodium: 420mg
- Carbohydrate: 6g
- Protein: 29g
- Fiber: 2g

Directions:

1. In a large salad bowl, combine the diced chicken, cucumber, cherry tomatoes, Kalamata olives, feta cheese, and red onion.

2. In a small bowl, whisk together the olive oil, red wine vinegar, dried oregano, salt, and pepper to create the dressing.

3. Pour the dressing over the salad and toss well to ensure all the ingredients are evenly coated.

4. Serve chilled or at room temperature. Enjoy a hearty and flavourful Greek salad that's perfect for a nutritious and satisfying meal.

Shrimp and Avocado Salad

Ingredients:

- 1 lb large shrimp, peeled and deveined
- 2 avocados, diced
- 1 cup cherry tomatoes, halved
- 1/4 cup red onion, finely chopped
- 1/4 cup cilantro, chopped

For the dressing:

- Juice of 2 limes
- 3 tablespoons olive oil
- 1 garlic clove, minced
- Salt and pepper to taste

Prep Time: 15 mins

Cooking Time: 5 mins

Total Time: 20 mins

Servings: 4

Nutrition Facts (per serving):

- Calories: 350
- Fat: 24g
- Saturated Fat: 3.5g
- Cholesterol: 180mg
- Sodium: 300mg
- Carbohydrate: 12g
- Protein: 24g
- Fiber: 7g

Directions:

1. Cook the shrimp in boiling water until pink and opaque, about 2-3 minutes. Drain and let cool.

2. In a large salad bowl, combine the cooled shrimp, diced avocados, cherry tomatoes, red onion, and cilantro.

3. In a small bowl, whisk together the lime juice, olive oil, minced garlic, salt, and pepper to create the dressing.

4. Pour the dressing over the salad and gently toss to combine.

5. Serve immediately, enjoying a vibrant and refreshing salad that's packed with protein and healthy fats.

Cobb Salad with Blue Cheese Dressing

Ingredients:

- 6 cups mixed salad greens
- 2 hard-boiled eggs, quartered
- 1 avocado, diced
- 1/2 cup cherry tomatoes, halved
- 1/2 cup cooked bacon, crumbled
- 1/2 cup blue cheese, crumbled
- 1/2 cup cooked chicken breast, diced

For the dressing:

- 1/2 cup Greek yogurt, full-fat
- 1/4 cup blue cheese, crumbled
- 2 tablespoons milk
- 1 tablespoon white wine vinegar
- Salt and pepper to taste

Prep Time: 20 mins

Cooking Time: 0 mins

Total Time: 20 mins

Servings: 4

Nutrition Facts (per serving):

- Calories: 400
- Fat: 30g
- Saturated Fat: 10g
- Cholesterol: 150mg
- Sodium: 620mg

- Carbohydrate: 8g
- Protein: 25g
- Fiber: 4g

Directions:

1. Arrange the mixed salad greens in a large serving bowl or platter.

2. Neatly arrange rows of hard-boiled eggs, diced avocado, cherry tomatoes, crumbled bacon, blue cheese, and diced chicken over the greens.

3. In a small bowl, mix together the Greek yogurt, blue cheese, milk, and white wine vinegar to create the dressing. Season with salt and pepper to taste.

4. Serve the salad with the blue cheese dressing on the side, allowing everyone to dress their salad to their liking. Enjoy a classic Cobb salad that's both delicious and aligned with a low-carb lifestyle.

Seared Scallops with Cauliflower Puree

Ingredients:

- 12 large sea scallops
- 1 head cauliflower, cut into florets
- 2 tablespoons olive oil
- 3 tablespoons unsalted butter
- 1/4 cup heavy cream
- Salt and pepper to taste
- Fresh chives, chopped for garnish
- Lemon wedges for serving

Prep Time: 10 mins

Cooking Time: 20 mins

Total Time: 30 mins

Servings: 4

Nutrition Facts (per serving):

- Calories: 290
- Fat: 22g
- Saturated Fat: 10g
- Cholesterol: 55mg
- Sodium: 320mg
- Carbohydrate: 10g
- Protein: 15g
- Fiber: 3g

Directions:

1. Steam cauliflower florets until very tender, about 15 minutes. Transfer to a blender, add heavy cream, 1 tablespoon butter, salt, and pepper. Blend until smooth.

2. Pat scallops dry with paper towels and season with salt and pepper. Heat olive oil in a large skillet over high heat. Add scallops, searing until a golden crust forms, about 2 minutes per side. Remove from skillet and set aside.

3. In the same skillet, melt the remaining 2 tablespoons of butter over medium heat. Add a squeeze of lemon juice.

4. To serve, spoon cauliflower puree onto plates, top with scallops, drizzle with lemon butter sauce, and garnish with chives. Serve with lemon wedges on the side.

Walnut-Crusted Salmon Salad

Ingredients:

- 4 salmon fillets (6 oz each)
- 1 cup walnuts, finely chopped
- 2 tablespoons Dijon mustard
- 8 cups mixed greens

- 1/2 cup cherry tomatoes, halved
- 1/4 cup red onion, thinly sliced

For the dressing:

- 3 tablespoons olive oil
- 2 tablespoons balsamic vinegar
- 1 teaspoon honey (optional, for low-carb, use a sugar-free substitute)
- Salt and pepper to taste

Prep Time: 15 mins

Cooking Time: 15 mins

Total Time: 30 mins

Servings: 4

Nutrition Facts (per serving):

- Calories: 510
- Fat: 38g
- Saturated Fat: 5g
- Cholesterol: 95mg
- Sodium: 200mg
- Carbohydrate: 10g
- Protein: 35g
- Fiber: 4g

Directions:

1. Preheat oven to 400°F (200°C). Spread walnuts on a plate. Brush each salmon fillet with Dijon mustard, then press into walnuts to coat.

2. Place salmon on a baking sheet lined with parchment paper. Bake until salmon is cooked through and walnuts are toasted, about 12-15 minutes.

3. While salmon bakes, whisk together olive oil, balsamic vinegar, honey, salt, and pepper to make the dressing.

4. Toss mixed greens, cherry tomatoes, and red onion with the dressing. Divide salad among plates.

5. Top each salad with a walnut-crusted salmon fillet. Serve immediately for a nutritious and satisfying meal.

Beef Taco Salad Bowl

Ingredients:

- 1 lb ground beef
- 1 tablespoon taco seasoning
- 4 cups romaine lettuce, chopped
- 1 avocado, diced
- 1/2 cup cherry tomatoes, halved
- 1/4 cup cheddar cheese, shredded
- 1/4 cup sour cream
- 1/4 cup salsa
- Fresh cilantro for garnish

Prep Time: 10 mins

Cooking Time: 10 mins

Total Time: 20 mins

Servings: 4

Nutrition Facts (per serving):

- Calories: 450
- Fat: 32g
- Saturated Fat: 12g
- Cholesterol: 100mg
- Sodium: 400mg
- Carbohydrate: 10g

- Protein: 32g
- Fiber: 5g

Directions:

1. Brown ground beef in a skillet over medium heat. Drain excess fat, then stir in taco seasoning and cook according to package instructions.

2. In serving bowls, layer chopped romaine lettuce, cooked taco-seasoned beef, diced avocado, cherry tomatoes, and shredded cheddar cheese.

3. Top each salad bowl with a dollop of sour cream and a spoonful of salsa. Garnish with fresh cilantro.

4. Serve immediately, allowing everyone to enjoy a deconstructed taco in salad form, perfect for a low-carb diet.

Mediterranean Chickpea Salad

Ingredients:

- 2 cans (15 oz each) chickpeas, drained and rinsed
- 1 cucumber, diced
- 1 bell pepper, diced
- 1/2 cup Kalamata olives, halved
- 1/2 cup feta cheese, crumbled
- 1/4 cup red onion, thinly sliced

For the dressing:

- 1/4 cup olive oil
- 2 tablespoons lemon juice
- 1 garlic clove, minced
- 1 teaspoon dried oregano
- Salt and pepper to taste

Prep Time: 15 mins

Cooking Time: 0 mins

Total Time: 15 mins

Servings: 4

Nutrition Facts (per serving):

- Calories: 360
- Fat: 20g
- Saturated Fat: 5g
- Cholesterol: 25mg
- Sodium: 720mg
- Carbohydrate: 34g
- Protein: 12g
- Fiber: 9g

Directions:

1. In a large bowl, combine chickpeas, cucumber, bell pepper, Kalamata olives, feta cheese, and red onion.

2. In a small bowl, whisk together olive oil, lemon juice, minced garlic, dried oregano, salt, and pepper to create the dressing.

3. Pour the dressing over the salad and toss to coat evenly.

4. Serve immediately or chill in the refrigerator for an hour to allow flavours to meld. Enjoy a refreshing and protein-packed Mediterranean salad.

Asian Cabbage Salad with Grilled Chicken

Ingredients:

- 2 cups cooked chicken breast, shredded
- 4 cups cabbage, shredded
- 1 carrot, julienned
- 1/2 cup red bell pepper, thinly sliced
- 1/4 cup green onions, sliced

- 1/4 cup almonds, sliced and toasted

For the dressing:

- 3 tablespoons soy sauce, low sodium
- 2 tablespoons rice vinegar
- 1 tablespoon sesame oil
- 1 tablespoon erythritol (or sweetener of choice)
- 1 teaspoon ginger, grated
- 1 garlic clove, minced

Prep Time: 20 mins

Cooking Time: 0 mins

Total Time: 20 mins

Servings: 4

Nutrition Facts (per serving):

- Calories: 250
- Fat: 12g
- Saturated Fat: 2g
- Cholesterol: 60mg
- Sodium: 430mg
- Carbohydrate: 10g
- Protein: 27g
- Fiber: 3g

Directions:

1. In a large salad bowl, combine shredded chicken, cabbage, carrot, red bell pepper, and green onions.

2. In a small bowl, whisk together soy sauce, rice vinegar, sesame oil, erythritol, ginger, and garlic to make the dressing.

3. Pour the dressing over the salad and toss well to ensure all ingredients are evenly coated.

4. Sprinkle toasted almonds over the top of the salad before serving.

5. Enjoy a crunchy and flavourful salad that's perfect for a light yet satisfying meal.

Grilled Portobello Mushroom Steaks

Ingredients:

- 4 large portobello mushrooms, stems removed
- 1/4 cup balsamic vinegar
- 2 tablespoons olive oil
- 2 cloves garlic, minced
- 1 teaspoon dried rosemary
- Salt and pepper to taste
- Fresh parsley, chopped for garnish

Prep Time: 10 mins (plus marinating time)

Cooking Time: 8 mins

Total Time: 18 mins (plus marinating time)

Servings: 4

Nutrition Facts (per serving):

- Calories: 120
- Fat: 7g
- Saturated Fat: 1g
- Cholesterol: 0mg
- Sodium: 15mg
- Carbohydrate: 11g
- Protein: 3g
- Fiber: 2g

Directions:

1. In a small bowl, whisk together balsamic vinegar, olive oil, minced garlic, dried rosemary, salt, and pepper.

2. Place portobello mushrooms in a large resealable plastic bag or shallow dish. Pour the marinade over the mushrooms, ensuring they are well coated. Marinate for at least 30 minutes, or up to 2 hours, turning occasionally.

3. Preheat grill to medium-high heat. Remove mushrooms from marinade, reserving excess marinade for basting.

4. Grill mushrooms for 4 minutes on each side, basting with reserved marinade, until tender and grill marks appear.

5. Serve hot, garnished with fresh parsley. Enjoy a delicious and hearty plant-based alternative to traditional steaks.

Crunchy Asian Slaw

Ingredients:

- 4 cups shredded cabbage (mix of green and red)
- 1 cup shredded carrots
- 1/2 cup thinly sliced red bell pepper
- 1/4 cup green onions, sliced
- 1/4 cup cilantro, chopped
- 1/2 cup slivered almonds, toasted

For the dressing:

- 3 tablespoons soy sauce, low sodium
- 2 tablespoons rice vinegar
- 1 tablespoon sesame oil
- 1 tablespoon peanut butter
- 1 tablespoon erythritol (or sweetener of choice)
- 1 teaspoon ginger, grated
- 1 clove garlic, minced

Prep Time: 15 mins

Cooking Time: 0 mins

Total Time: 15 mins

Servings: 4

Nutrition Facts (per serving):

- Calories: 180
- Fat: 12g
- Saturated Fat: 1.5g
- Cholesterol: 0mg
- Sodium: 430mg
- Carbohydrate: 14g
- Protein: 5g
- Fiber: 4g

Directions:

1. In a large salad bowl, combine shredded cabbage, carrots, red bell pepper, green onions, and cilantro.

2. In a small bowl, whisk together all the dressing ingredients until smooth and well combined.

3. Pour the dressing over the salad and toss to coat evenly.

4. Sprinkle toasted slivered almonds over the top before serving.

5. Enjoy a vibrant and crunchy salad that's bursting with flavours, perfect as a side dish or a light meal.

Lemon Garlic Butter Cod

Ingredients:

- 4 cod fillets (6 oz each)
- 2 tablespoons butter
- 2 cloves garlic, minced

- Juice and zest of 1 lemon

- 1 tablespoon fresh parsley, chopped

- Salt and pepper to taste

Prep Time: 5 mins

Cooking Time: 12 mins

Total Time: 17 mins

Servings: 4

Nutrition Facts (per serving):

- Calories: 190

- Fat: 7g

- Saturated Fat: 4g

- Cholesterol: 75mg

- Sodium: 125mg

- Carbohydrate: 1g

- Protein: 30g

- Fiber: 0g

Directions:

1. Season cod fillets with salt and pepper. Heat butter in a large skillet over medium heat.

2. Add garlic to the skillet and sauté until fragrant, about 1 minute.

3. Place cod fillets in the skillet and cook for 5-6 minutes on each side, or until the fish flakes easily with a fork.

4. Drizzle lemon juice over the cod during the last minute of cooking. Sprinkle with lemon zest and fresh parsley before serving.

5. Enjoy a simple yet elegant fish dish that's full of flavor and perfect for a healthy dinner.

Roasted Vegetable Quinoa Salad

Ingredients:

- 1 cup quinoa, rinsed
- 2 cups vegetable broth
- 2 cups mixed vegetables (zucchini, bell peppers, cherry tomatoes), chopped
- 2 tablespoons olive oil
- Salt and pepper to taste
- 1/4 cup feta cheese, crumbled
- 1/4 cup fresh basil, chopped

For the dressing:

- 3 tablespoons olive oil
- 2 tablespoons lemon juice
- 1 teaspoon Dijon mustard
- Salt and pepper to taste

Prep Time: 10 mins

Cooking Time: 25 mins

Total Time: 35 mins

Servings: 4

Nutrition Facts (per serving):

- Calories: 350
- Fat: 18g
- Saturated Fat: 3g
- Cholesterol: 8mg
- Sodium: 320mg
- Carbohydrate: 38g
- Protein: 10g
- Fiber: 5g

Directions:

1. Preheat oven to 425°F (220°C). Toss chopped vegetables with 2 tablespoons olive oil, salt, and pepper. Spread on a baking sheet and roast for 20 minutes, until tender and caramelized.

2. Meanwhile, bring vegetable broth to a boil in a medium saucepan. Add quinoa, reduce heat to low, cover, and simmer for 15 minutes, or until liquid is absorbed.

3. Fluff quinoa with a fork and transfer to a large salad bowl. Add roasted vegetables, feta cheese, and fresh basil.

4. In a small bowl, whisk together dressing ingredients. Pour over the salad and toss to combine.

5. Serve warm or at room temperature. Enjoy a nutritious and satisfying salad that's perfect for a light lunch or dinner.

Spicy Avocado Egg Salad

Ingredients:

- 6 hard-boiled eggs, peeled and chopped
- 2 ripe avocados, mashed
- 1/4 cup mayonnaise, low carb
- 1 tablespoon Dijon mustard
- 1 jalapeño, seeded and finely chopped
- 2 tablespoons red onion, finely chopped
- 2 tablespoons cilantro, chopped
- Juice of 1 lime
- Salt and pepper to taste

Prep Time: 15 mins

Cooking Time: 0 mins

Total Time: 15 mins

Servings: 4

- Calories: 300
- Fat: 25g
- Saturated Fat: 5g
- Cholesterol: 280mg
- Sodium: 220mg
- Carbohydrate: 8g
- Protein: 12g
- Fiber: 5g

Directions:

1. In a large bowl, combine chopped hard-boiled eggs and mashed avocados.

2. Stir in mayonnaise, Dijon mustard, jalapeño, red onion, cilantro, and lime juice. Mix well until all ingredients are evenly incorporated.

3. Season with salt and pepper to taste.

4. Serve immediately or chill in the refrigerator for an hour to allow flavours to meld. Enjoy a creamy and spicy twist on the classic egg salad, perfect for sandwiches or as a dip with low-carb crackers.

Creamy Tuscan Garlic Chicken

Ingredients:

- 4 boneless, skinless chicken breasts
- Salt and pepper to taste
- 2 tablespoons olive oil
- 1 cup heavy cream
- 1/2 cup chicken broth
- 1 teaspoon garlic powder
- 1 teaspoon Italian seasoning

- 1/2 cup sun-dried tomatoes, chopped
- 1 cup spinach, chopped
- 1/2 cup grated Parmesan cheese

Prep Time: 10 mins

Cooking Time: 20 mins

Total Time: 30 mins

Servings: 4

Nutrition Facts (per serving):

- Calories: 450
- Fat: 30g
- Saturated Fat: 15g
- Cholesterol: 145mg
- Sodium: 390mg
- Carbohydrate: 8g
- Protein: 38g
- Fiber: 1g

Directions:

1. Season chicken breasts with salt and pepper. Heat olive oil in a large skillet over medium-high heat. Add chicken and cook until golden and cooked through, about 6-8 minutes per side. Remove chicken and set aside.

2. In the same skillet, add heavy cream, chicken broth, garlic powder, and Italian seasoning. Whisk to combine and bring to a simmer. Add sun-dried tomatoes and spinach, simmering until the spinach wilts, about 2-3 minutes.

3. Stir in Parmesan cheese until melted and sauce is creamy. Return chicken to the skillet and spoon the sauce over the chicken.

4. Serve hot, garnished with additional Parmesan or fresh herbs if desired. Enjoy a rich and flavorful dish that's perfect for a comforting dinner.

Zesty Lime Shrimp and Avocado Salad

Ingredients:

- 1 lb shrimp, peeled and deveined
- 2 avocados, diced
- 1/4 cup red onion, finely chopped
- 2 limes, juiced
- 1 teaspoon zest from lime
- 1/4 cup cilantro, chopped
- Salt and pepper to taste
- 1 jalapeño, seeded and finely chopped (optional)

Prep Time: 15 mins

Cooking Time: 5 mins

Total Time: 20 mins

Servings: 4

Nutrition Facts (per serving):

- Calories: 290
- Fat: 18g
- Saturated Fat: 3g
- Cholesterol: 180mg
- Sodium: 210mg
- Carbohydrate: 10g
- Protein: 25g
- Fiber: 7g

Directions:

1. Cook shrimp in boiling water until pink and opaque, about 2-3 minutes. Drain and let cool.

2. In a large bowl, combine cooled shrimp, diced avocados, red onion, lime juice, lime zest, cilantro, salt, and pepper. Add jalapeño if using for extra spice.

3. Gently toss to combine all ingredients. Adjust seasoning to taste.

4. Chill in the refrigerator for 10 minutes before serving to allow flavours to meld.

5. Serve as a refreshing and light salad, perfect for a quick lunch or as an appetizer.

Roasted Brussels Sprouts and Bacon

Ingredients:

- 1 lb Brussels sprouts, trimmed and halved
- 6 slices bacon, chopped
- 2 tablespoons olive oil
- Salt and pepper to taste
- 2 tablespoons balsamic vinegar (optional)

Prep Time: 10 mins

Cooking Time: 25 mins

Total Time: 35 mins

Servings: 4

Nutrition Facts (per serving):

- Calories: 250
- Fat: 18g
- Saturated Fat: 5g
- Cholesterol: 25mg
- Sodium: 300mg
- Carbohydrate: 12g
- Protein: 10g

- Fiber: 4g

Directions:

1. Preheat oven to 400°F (200°C). On a large baking sheet, toss Brussels sprouts and chopped bacon with olive oil, salt, and pepper until well coated.

2. Spread the Brussels sprouts and bacon in a single layer and roast in the preheated oven for 20-25 minutes, until Brussels sprouts are tender and caramelized, and bacon is crispy.

3. Drizzle with balsamic vinegar and toss to coat evenly (optional).

4. Serve hot as a delicious side dish that pairs well with any main course, offering a perfect combination of savoury flavours and crispy textures.

Cauliflower and Cheese Stuffed Peppers

Ingredients:

- 4 large bell peppers, halved and seeded
- 1 head cauliflower, riced
- 1 cup sharp cheddar cheese, shredded
- 1/2 cup cream cheese, softened
- 1/4 cup green onions, chopped
- Salt and pepper to taste
- 1/2 teaspoon paprika
- 1/4 cup Parmesan cheese, for topping

Prep Time: 15 mins

Cooking Time: 25 mins

Total Time: 40 mins

Servings: 4

Nutrition Facts (per serving):

- Calories: 320

- Fat: 22g
- Saturated Fat: 13g
- Cholesterol: 60mg
- Sodium: 420mg
- Carbohydrate: 15g
- Protein: 18g
- Fiber: 4g

Directions:

1. Preheat oven to 375°F (190°C). Place bell pepper halves in a baking dish, cut-side up.

2. In a large bowl, mix together riced cauliflower, sharp cheddar cheese, cream cheese, green onions, salt, pepper, and paprika until well combined.

3. Spoon the cauliflower mixture into each bell pepper half, pressing down to fill completely.

4. Sprinkle the tops of the stuffed peppers with Parmesan cheese.

5. Bake in the preheated oven for 25 minutes, or until the peppers are tender and the tops are golden brown.

6. Serve warm as a hearty and flavorful vegetarian dish that's both satisfying and low in carbs.

Spicy Tuna and Avocado Cucumber Cups

Ingredients:

- 2 large cucumbers, sliced into thick rounds
- 1 can (5 oz) tuna in water, drained
- 1 ripe avocado, mashed, 1 tablespoon mayonnaise, low carb
- 1 teaspoon Sriracha sauce (adjust to taste)
- 1/4 cup cilantro, chopped
- Salt and pepper to taste

- Sesame seeds for garnish

Prep Time: 20 mins

Cooking Time: 0 mins

Total Time: 20 mins

Servings: 4

Nutrition Facts (per serving):

- Calories: 150

- Fat: 10g

- Saturated Fat: 1.5g

- Cholesterol: 15mg

- Sodium: 180mg

- Carbohydrate: 7g

- Protein: 9g

- Fiber: 4g

Directions:

1. Using a melon baller or small spoon, scoop out the center of each cucumber round to create a cup, leaving the bottom intact.

2. In a bowl, mix together the drained tuna, mashed avocado, mayonnaise, Sriracha sauce, cilantro, salt, and pepper until well combined.

3. Spoon the tuna mixture into the cucumber cups, filling them generously.

4. Sprinkle sesame seeds over the top of each cucumber cup for garnish.

5. Serve immediately as a refreshing and spicy appetizer or snack, perfect for a healthy and low-carb option at any gathering

SNACK RECIPES

Cheesy Cauliflower Breadsticks

Ingredients:

- 1 head cauliflower, riced
- 1 egg, beaten
- 1 cup mozzarella cheese, shredded (divided)
- 2 teaspoons garlic, minced
- 1/2 teaspoon dried oregano
- Salt and pepper to taste
- Marinara sauce for dipping (optional)

Prep Time: 15 mins

Cooking Time: 25 mins

Total Time: 40 mins

Servings: 4

Nutrition Facts (per serving):

- Calories: 150
- Fat: 8g
- Saturated Fat: 4g
- Cholesterol: 60mg
- Sodium: 200mg
- Carbohydrate: 8g
- Protein: 12g
- Fiber: 3g

Directions:

1. Preheat oven to 425°F (220°C). Line a baking sheet with parchment paper.

2. Microwave riced cauliflower for 5 minutes. Let it cool, then squeeze out as much moisture as possible using a clean kitchen towel.

3. In a bowl, combine the drained cauliflower, egg, 1/2 cup mozzarella, garlic, oregano, salt, and pepper. Mix well.

4. Spread the cauliflower mixture onto the prepared baking sheet, forming a rectangle about 1/4 inch thick.

5. Bake for 20 minutes, or until golden. Sprinkle the remaining 1/2 cup mozzarella over the top and return to the oven for an additional 5 minutes, until cheese is melted and bubbly.

6. Cut into sticks and serve warm with marinara sauce for dipping. Enjoy a delicious and low-carb alternative to traditional breadsticks.

Avocado Chocolate Mousse

Ingredients:

- 2 ripe avocados, peeled and pitted
- 1/4 cup cocoa powder
- 1/4 cup almond milk
- 1/4 cup erythritol (or sweetener of choice)
- 1 teaspoon vanilla extract
- Pinch of salt
- Whipped cream for topping (optional)

Prep Time: 10 mins

Cooking Time: 0 mins

Total Time: 10 mins

Servings: 4

Nutrition Facts (per serving):

- Calories: 200
- Fat: 15g

- Saturated Fat: 2g
- Cholesterol: 0mg
- Sodium: 40mg
- Carbohydrate: 12g
- Protein: 3g
- Fiber: 7g

Directions:

1. In a blender or food processor, combine avocados, cocoa powder, almond milk, erythritol, vanilla extract, and a pinch of salt. Blend until smooth and creamy.

2. Divide the mousse into serving dishes and refrigerate for at least 1 hour to chill and set.

3. Serve topped with whipped cream if desired. Enjoy a rich and creamy chocolate mousse that's not only delicious but also healthy and low in carbs.

Spicy Roasted Almonds

Ingredients:

- 2 cups raw almonds
- 1 tablespoon olive oil, 1 teaspoon chili powder
- 1/2 teaspoon cumin
- 1/2 teaspoon garlic powder
- Salt to taste

Prep Time: 5 mins

Cooking Time: 15 mins

Total Time: 20 mins

Servings: 8

Nutrition Facts (per serving):

- Calories: 170

- Fat: 15g

- Saturated Fat: 1g

- Cholesterol: 0mg

- Sodium: 75mg

- Carbohydrate: 6g

- Protein: 6g

- Fiber: 3g

Directions:

1. Preheat oven to 350°F (175°C). Line a baking sheet with parchment paper.

2. In a bowl, toss almonds with olive oil, chili powder, cumin, garlic powder, and salt until well coated.

3. Spread almonds in a single layer on the prepared baking sheet.

4. Roast in the preheated oven for 15 minutes, stirring halfway through, until golden and fragrant.

5. Let cool before serving. Enjoy a spicy and savory snack that's perfect for satisfying hunger between meals.

Cucumber Roll-Ups with Hummus

Ingredients:

- 2 large cucumbers

- 1 cup hummus

- 1/4 cup red bell pepper, finely diced

- 1/4 cup carrot, finely diced

- 1/4 cup spinach, chopped

- Salt and pepper to taste

Prep Time: 20 mins

Cooking Time: 0 mins

Total Time: 20 mins

Servings: 4

Nutrition Facts (per serving):

- Calories: 120
- Fat: 7g
- Saturated Fat: 1g
- Cholesterol: 0mg
- Sodium: 300mg
- Carbohydrate: 12g
- Protein: 5g
- Fiber: 4g

Directions:

1. Use a vegetable peeler or mandolin slicer to cut the cucumbers into long, thin slices.
2. Lay cucumber slices on a clean surface and pat dry with paper towels.
3. Spread a thin layer of hummus over each cucumber slice.
4. Sprinkle red bell pepper, carrot, and spinach evenly over the hummus-covered cucumber slices.
5. Carefully roll up the cucumber slices tightly.
6. Serve immediately or chill in the refrigerator before serving. Enjoy a refreshing and healthy snack that's perfect for a quick bite or as a party appetizer.

Mini Bell Pepper Nachos

Ingredients:

- 8 mini bell peppers, halved and seeded
- 1 cup cooked ground turkey or beef
- 1 teaspoon taco seasoning

- 1/2 cup cheddar cheese, shredded
- 1/4 cup black olives, sliced
- 1/4 cup cherry tomatoes, diced
- 1/4 cup green onions, chopped
- Sour cream and salsa for serving

Prep Time: 10 mins

Cooking Time: 10 mins

Total Time: 20 mins

Servings: 4

Nutrition Facts (per serving):

- Calories: 180
- Fat: 10g
- Saturated Fat: 4g
- Cholesterol: 40mg
- Sodium: 220mg
- Carbohydrate: 8g
- Protein: 15g
- Fiber: 2g

Directions:

1. Preheat oven to 375°F (190°C). Arrange mini bell pepper halves on a baking sheet, cut-side up.

2. In a bowl, mix cooked ground turkey or beef with taco seasoning. Spoon the mixture into each bell pepper half.

3. Sprinkle shredded cheddar cheese over the top of each stuffed pepper.

4. Bake in the preheated oven for 10 minutes, or until the cheese is melted and bubbly.

5. Garnish with black olives, diced cherry tomatoes, and green onions.

6. Serve with sour cream and salsa on the side. Enjoy a low-carb take on traditional nachos, perfect for a healthy snack or appetizer.

Smoked Salmon and Cream Cheese Cucumber Bites

Ingredients:

- 2 large cucumbers, sliced into rounds
- 8 oz cream cheese, softened
- 4 oz smoked salmon, cut into bite-size pieces
- 1 tablespoon fresh dill, chopped
- 1 tablespoon capers, drained
- Black pepper to taste

Prep Time: 15 mins

Cooking Time: 0 mins

Total Time: 15 mins

Servings: 6

Nutrition Facts (per serving):

- Calories: 150
- Fat: 12g
- Saturated Fat: 7g
- Cholesterol: 40mg
- Sodium: 300mg
- Carbohydrate: 3g
- Protein: 7g
- Fiber: 1g

Directions:

1. Arrange cucumber slices on a serving platter.

2. In a bowl, mix cream cheese until smooth. Spread a thin layer of cream cheese on each cucumber slice.

3. Top each cucumber round with a piece of smoked salmon. Sprinkle with fresh dill, capers, and a touch of black pepper.

4. Serve immediately or chill in the refrigerator for up to an hour before serving. Enjoy a refreshing and elegant snack perfect for gatherings or a light appetizer.

Keto Jalapeño Poppers

Ingredients:

- 12 jalapeño peppers, halved lengthwise and seeded
- 8 oz cream cheese, softened
- 1 cup cheddar cheese, shredded
- 1/2 teaspoon garlic powder
- 1/2 teaspoon onion powder
- 12 slices of bacon, cut in half

Prep Time: 20 mins

Cooking Time: 20 mins

Total Time: 40 mins

Servings: 6

Nutrition Facts (per serving):

- Calories: 320
- Fat: 28g
- Saturated Fat: 13g
- Cholesterol: 75mg
- Sodium: 500mg
- Carbohydrate: 4g
- Protein: 15g
- Fiber: 1g

Directions:

1. Preheat oven to 400°F (200°C). Line a baking sheet with parchment paper.

2. In a bowl, mix together cream cheese, cheddar cheese, garlic powder, and onion powder until well combined.

3. Fill each jalapeño half with the cheese mixture.

4. Wrap a half slice of bacon around each stuffed jalapeño half and place on the prepared baking sheet.

5. Bake in the preheated oven for 20 minutes or until bacon is crispy and peppers are tender.

6. Serve hot as a spicy and creamy snack that's sure to be a hit at any party or gathering.

Prosciutto-Wrapped Asparagus

Ingredients:

- 16 asparagus spears, trimmed
- 8 slices of prosciutto, cut in half lengthwise
- 1 tablespoon olive oil
- Black pepper to taste
- Parmesan cheese, shaved (optional)

Prep Time: 10 mins

Cooking Time: 15 mins

Total Time: 25 mins

Servings: 4

Nutrition Facts (per serving):

- Calories: 120
- Fat: 8g
- Saturated Fat: 2g
- Cholesterol: 20mg

- Sodium: 320mg

- Carbohydrate: 3g

- Protein: 10g

- Fiber: 1g

Directions:

1. Preheat oven to 400°F (200°C). Line a baking sheet with parchment paper.

2. Wrap each asparagus spear with a half slice of prosciutto, leaving the tips exposed.

3. Arrange wrapped asparagus on the baking sheet. Drizzle with olive oil and sprinkle with black pepper.

4. Bake in the preheated oven for 15 minutes, or until asparagus is tender and prosciutto is crispy.

5. Serve garnished with shaved Parmesan cheese if desired. Enjoy a simple yet sophisticated snack that pairs perfectly with your favourite low-carb dip or sauce.

Greek Yogurt Berry Parfait

Ingredients:

- 2 cups Greek yogurt, full-fat

- 1 cup mixed berries (strawberries, blueberries, raspberries)

- 1/4 cup almonds, sliced and toasted

- 2 tablespoons erythritol (or sweetener of choice)

- 1 teaspoon vanilla extract

Prep Time: 10 mins

Cooking Time: 0 mins

Total Time: 10 mins

Servings: 4

Nutrition Facts (per serving):

- Calories: 180

- Fat: 9g

- Saturated Fat: 3g

- Cholesterol: 10mg

- Sodium: 50mg

- Carbohydrate: 10g

- Protein: 15g

- Fiber: 2g

Directions:

1. In a bowl, mix Greek yogurt with erythritol and vanilla extract until well combined.

2. In serving glasses or bowls, layer Greek yogurt mixture, mixed berries, and toasted almonds.

3. Repeat the layers until all ingredients are used up, finishing with a layer of berries and almonds on top.

4. Serve immediately or chill in the refrigerator for a refreshing and nutritious snack that's both satisfying and low in carbs.

Cheesy Zucchini Bites

Ingredients:

- 2 medium zucchinis, grated

- 1 egg, beaten

- 1/2 cup almond flour

- 1/2 cup Parmesan cheese, grated

- 1/2 teaspoon garlic powder

- Salt and pepper to taste

- 1/4 cup mozzarella cheese, shredded for topping

Prep Time: 15 mins

Cooking Time: 20 mins

Total Time: 35 mins

Servings: 4

Nutrition Facts (per serving):

- Calories: 180
- Fat: 12g
- Saturated Fat: 4g
- Cholesterol: 60mg
- Sodium: 320mg
- Carbohydrate: 6g
- Protein: 12g
- Fiber: 2g

Directions:

1. Preheat oven to 400°F (200°C). Line a baking sheet with parchment paper.

2. Squeeze excess moisture out of the grated zucchini using a clean kitchen towel.

3. In a bowl, combine zucchini, egg, almond flour, Parmesan cheese, garlic powder, salt, and pepper. Mix well to form a sticky dough.

4. Shape the mixture into small bite-sized balls and place on the prepared baking sheet. Flatten slightly with the back of a spoon.

5. Sprinkle shredded mozzarella cheese on top of each zucchini bite.

6. Bake in the preheated oven for 20 minutes, or until golden and crispy.

7. Serve hot as a delicious and healthy snack that's perfect for satisfying those savoury cravings.

Eggplant Chips with Tzatziki Dip

Ingredients:

- 2 large eggplants, thinly sliced
- 2 tablespoons olive oil
- 1 teaspoon sea salt
- 1/2 teaspoon black pepper
- 1/2 teaspoon smoked paprika

For the Tzatziki Dip:

- 1 cup Greek yogurt, full-fat
- 1 small cucumber, grated and drained
- 2 cloves garlic, minced
- 2 tablespoons fresh dill, chopped
- 1 tablespoon lemon juice
- Salt and pepper to taste

Prep Time: 15 mins

Cooking Time: 25 mins

Total Time: 40 mins

Servings: 4

Nutrition Facts (per serving):

- Calories: 150
- Fat: 8g
- Saturated Fat: 2g
- Cholesterol: 5mg
- Sodium: 620mg
- Carbohydrate: 12g
- Protein: 6g
- Fiber: 5g

Directions:

1. Preheat oven to 375°F (190°C). Line two baking sheets with parchment paper.

2. Toss eggplant slices with olive oil, sea salt, pepper, and smoked paprika until evenly coated.

3. Arrange eggplant slices in a single layer on the baking sheets. Bake for 20-25 minutes, flipping halfway through, until crispy and golden.

4. While the eggplant is baking, prepare the tzatziki dip by combining Greek yogurt, grated cucumber, minced garlic, chopped dill, lemon juice, salt, and pepper in a bowl. Mix well and refrigerate until serving.

5. Serve the crispy eggplant chips with the chilled tzatziki dip. Enjoy a healthy and flavourful snack that's perfect for sharing.

Spicy Buffalo Cauliflower Bites

Ingredients:

- 1 head cauliflower, cut into bite-sized florets
- 1/2 cup almond flour
- 1/2 cup water
- 1 teaspoon garlic powder
- Salt and pepper to taste
- 1/2 cup hot sauce
- 2 tablespoons butter, melted

Prep Time: 10 mins

Cooking Time: 20 mins

Total Time: 30 mins

Servings: 4

Nutrition Facts (per serving):

- Calories: 160
- Fat: 10g

- Saturated Fat: 4g

- Cholesterol: 15mg

- Sodium: 1100mg

- Carbohydrate: 10g

- Protein: 4g

- Fiber: 4g

Directions:

1. Preheat oven to 450°F (230°C). Line a baking sheet with parchment paper.

2. In a bowl, mix almond flour, water, garlic powder, salt, and pepper to create a batter.

3. Dip cauliflower florets into the batter, ensuring each piece is well coated. Arrange on the baking sheet in a single layer.

4. Bake for 15 minutes, until the batter starts to harden.

5. In a separate bowl, combine hot sauce and melted butter.

6. Remove cauliflower from the oven and toss with the hot sauce mixture. Return to the oven and bake for an additional 5-10 minutes, until crispy.

7. Serve hot as a spicy and satisfying snack that's perfect for game day or any gathering.

Keto Avocado Fries

Ingredients:

- 2 ripe avocados, sliced into wedges

- 1/2 cup almond flour

- 1/4 cup coconut flour

- 1 teaspoon paprika

- Salt and pepper to taste

- 2 eggs, beaten

- 1/2 cup grated Parmesan cheese

Prep Time: 15 mins

Cooking Time: 15 mins

Total Time: 30 mins

Servings: 4

Nutrition Facts (per serving):

- Calories: 320

- Fat: 25g

- Saturated Fat: 7g

- Cholesterol: 105mg

- Sodium: 300mg

- Carbohydrate: 14g

- Protein: 13g

- Fiber: 9g

Directions:

1. Preheat oven to 400°F (200°C). Line a baking sheet with parchment paper.

2. In a shallow dish, combine almond flour, coconut flour, paprika, salt, and pepper.

3. Dip each avocado wedge first in the beaten eggs, then in the flour mixture, ensuring they are well coated.

4. Arrange the coated avocado wedges on the prepared baking sheet. Sprinkle with grated Parmesan cheese.

5. Bake for 15 minutes, or until the coating is crispy and golden.

6. Serve hot as a delicious and nutritious keto-friendly snack.

Peanut Butter Protein Balls

Ingredients:

- 1 cup natural peanut butter

- 1/4 cup coconut flour
- 2 tablespoons erythritol (or sweetener of choice)
- 1/2 cup protein powder (vanilla or chocolate)
- 1/4 cup almond milk
- 1/4 cup dark chocolate chips (sugar-free)

Prep Time: 10 mins

Cooking Time: 0 mins

Total Time: 10 mins (plus chilling time)

Servings: 8

Nutrition Facts (per serving):

- Calories: 280
- Fat: 18g
- Saturated Fat: 5g
- Cholesterol: 0mg
- Sodium: 150mg
- Carbohydrate: 10g
- Protein: 20g
- Fiber: 4g

Directions:

1. In a large bowl, mix together peanut butter, coconut flour, erythritol, and protein powder. Gradually add almond milk until the mixture reaches a dough-like consistency.

2. Fold in dark chocolate chips.

3. Roll the mixture into bite-sized balls and place on a baking sheet lined with parchment paper.

4. Refrigerate for at least 30 minutes to set.

5. Enjoy a protein-packed snack that's perfect for a post-workout boost or a midday treat.

Stuffed Mini Peppers with Goat Cheese

Ingredients:

- 12 mini bell peppers, halved and seeded
- 4 oz goat cheese, softened
- 2 tablespoons cream cheese, softened
- 1 tablespoon fresh chives, chopped
- Salt and pepper to taste
- 1/4 cup walnuts, chopped (optional)

Prep Time: 15 mins

Cooking Time: 0 mins

Total Time: 15 mins

Servings: 4

Nutrition Facts (per serving):

- Calories: 180
- Fat: 14g
- Saturated Fat: 7g
- Cholesterol: 20mg
- Sodium: 220mg
- Carbohydrate: 6g
- Protein: 7g
- Fiber: 2g

Directions:

1. In a bowl, mix together goat cheese, cream cheese, chives, salt, and pepper until smooth.

2. Carefully fill each mini pepper half with the cheese mixture, using a spoon or a piping bag for ease.

3. Sprinkle chopped walnuts over the filled peppers for added crunch (optional).

4. Serve immediately or chill in the refrigerator before serving. Enjoy a colourful and tasty snack that's both visually appealing and delicious.

Coconut Flour Pancakes

Ingredients:

- 1/2 cup coconut flour
- 4 large eggs
- 3/4 cup almond milk
- 2 tablespoons erythritol (or sweetener of choice)
- 1 teaspoon baking powder
- 1/2 teaspoon vanilla extract
- Pinch of salt
- Butter or coconut oil for frying

Prep Time: 10 mins

Cooking Time: 15 mins

Total Time: 25 mins

Servings: 4

Nutrition Facts (per serving):

- Calories: 180
- Fat: 10g
- Saturated Fat: 6g
- Cholesterol: 185mg
- Sodium: 220mg
- Carbohydrate: 9g
- Protein: 9g
- Fiber: 5g

Directions:

1. In a large bowl, whisk together coconut flour, eggs, almond milk, erythritol, baking powder, vanilla extract, and a pinch of salt until smooth.

2. Heat a non-stick skillet or griddle over medium heat and grease lightly with butter or coconut oil.

3. Pour 1/4 cup of batter for each pancake onto the skillet. Cook until bubbles form on the surface, then flip and cook until golden brown on the other side.

4. Serve hot with your favourite low-carb syrup or fresh berries. Enjoy a delicious and fluffy pancake breakfast that's both satisfying and low in carbs.

Zucchini Lasagna Roll-Ups

Ingredients:

- 4 large zucchinis, sliced lengthwise into thin strips
- 1 cup ricotta cheese
- 1/4 cup grated Parmesan cheese
- 1 large egg
- 1 cup spinach, chopped
- 2 cups marinara sauce, low carb
- 1 cup mozzarella cheese, shredded
- Salt and pepper to taste
- Fresh basil for garnish

Prep Time: 20 mins

Cooking Time: 25 mins

Total Time: 45 mins

Servings: 4

Nutrition Facts (per serving):

- Calories: 290
- Fat: 16g
- Saturated Fat: 9g
- Cholesterol: 95mg

- Sodium: 680mg

- Carbohydrate: 14g

- Protein: 23g

- Fiber: 3g

Directions:

1. Preheat oven to 375°F (190°C). Lay zucchini slices on paper towels, sprinkle with salt, and let sit for 10 minutes to draw out moisture. Pat dry.

2. In a bowl, mix ricotta cheese, Parmesan cheese, egg, chopped spinach, salt, and pepper.

3. Spread a thin layer of marinara sauce on the bottom of a baking dish.

4. Take a slice of zucchini and spread a layer of the ricotta mixture over it, then roll up and place seam side down in the baking dish. Repeat with remaining zucchini slices.

5. Pour the remaining marinara sauce over the roll-ups and sprinkle with shredded mozzarella cheese.

6. Bake in the preheated oven for 25 minutes, or until the cheese is bubbly and golden.

7. Garnish with fresh basil before serving. Enjoy a comforting and healthy twist on traditional lasagna that's perfect for a cozy dinner.

Spiced Nuts Mix

Ingredients:

- 2 cups mixed nuts (almonds, walnuts, pecans)

- 1 tablespoon olive oil

- 1 teaspoon ground cumin

- 1/2 teaspoon chili powder

- 1/2 teaspoon smoked paprika

- 1/4 teaspoon cayenne pepper (optional)

- Salt to taste

Prep Time: 5 mins

Cooking Time: 10 mins

Total Time: 15 mins

Servings: 8

Nutrition Facts (per serving):

- Calories: 210

- Fat: 19g

- Saturated Fat: 2g

- Cholesterol: 0mg

- Sodium: 75mg

- Carbohydrate: 7g

- Protein: 6g

- Fiber: 3g

Directions:

1. Preheat oven to 350°F (175°C). Line a baking sheet with parchment paper.

2. In a bowl, toss mixed nuts with olive oil, ground cumin, chili powder, smoked paprika, cayenne pepper, and salt until well coated.

3. Spread the nuts in a single layer on the prepared baking sheet.

4. Bake in the preheated oven for 10 minutes, stirring halfway through, until nuts are toasted and fragrant.

5. Let cool before serving. Enjoy a spicy and savoury snack that's perfect for munching on the go or serving at parties.

Creamy Avocado Dip

Ingredients:

- 2 ripe avocados, peeled and pitted

- 1/2 cup Greek yogurt, full-fat
- 1 clove garlic, minced
- 2 tablespoons lime juice
- 1/4 teaspoon cumin
- Salt and pepper to taste
- Fresh cilantro, chopped for garnish
- Red pepper flakes for garnish (optional)

Prep Time: 10 mins

Cooking Time: 0 mins

Total Time: 10 mins

Servings: 4

Nutrition Facts (per serving):

- Calories: 220
- Fat: 18g
- Saturated Fat: 3g
- Cholesterol: 5mg
- Sodium: 45mg
- Carbohydrate: 12g
- Protein: 4g
- Fiber: 7g

Directions:

1. In a food processor or blender, combine avocados, Greek yogurt, minced garlic, lime juice, cumin, salt, and pepper. Blend until smooth and creamy.

2. Transfer to a serving bowl and garnish with chopped cilantro and red pepper flakes if desired.

3. Serve with low-carb vegetables or keto-friendly crackers for dipping. Enjoy a creamy and flavourful dip that's perfect for any occasion.

Bacon-Wrapped Asparagus Bundles

Ingredients:

- 16 asparagus spears, trimmed
- 8 slices of bacon
- 1 tablespoon olive oil
- Salt and pepper to taste
- 1/4 teaspoon garlic powder

Prep Time: 10 mins

Cooking Time: 20 mins

Total Time: 30 mins

Servings: 4

Nutrition Facts (per serving):

- Calories: 180
- Fat: 15g
- Saturated Fat: 4g
- Cholesterol: 20mg
- Sodium: 300mg
- Carbohydrate: 3g
- Protein: 10g
- Fiber: 1g

Directions:

1. Preheat oven to 400°F (200°C). Line a baking sheet with parchment paper.

2. Wrap a slice of bacon around two asparagus spears to form a bundle. Repeat with the remaining asparagus and bacon.

3. Arrange the asparagus bundles on the prepared baking sheet. Drizzle with olive oil and season with salt, pepper, and garlic powder.

4. Bake in the preheated oven for 20 minutes, or until the bacon is crispy and asparagus is tender.

5. Serve hot as a delicious and elegant snack or side dish that's sure to impress.

DESSERT RECIPES

Keto Chocolate Avocado Pudding

Ingredients:

- 2 ripe avocados, peeled and pitted
- 1/4 cup unsweetened cocoa powder
- 1/4 cup almond milk
- 1/3 cup erythritol (or sweetener of choice)
- 1 teaspoon vanilla extract
- Pinch of salt

Prep Time: 10 mins

Cooking Time: 0 mins

Total Time: 10 mins

Servings: 4

Nutrition Facts (per serving):

- Calories: 160
- Fat: 12g
- Saturated Fat: 2g
- Cholesterol: 0mg
- Sodium: 40mg
- Carbohydrate: 12g
- Protein: 3g
- Fiber: 7g

Directions:

1. In a blender or food processor, combine avocados, cocoa powder, almond milk, erythritol, vanilla extract, and a pinch of salt. Blend until smooth and creamy.

2. Divide the pudding into serving dishes and refrigerate for at least 1 hour to chill and thicken.

3. Serve as a rich and creamy dessert that satisfies chocolate cravings without the carbs.

Almond Flour Lemon Bars

Ingredients:

For the crust:

- 1 1/2 cups almond flour
- 1/4 cup erythritol
- 1/4 cup unsalted butter, melted
- 1 teaspoon vanilla extract

For the filling:

- 3 eggs, 1/2 cup erythritol
- 1/2 cup lemon juice
- 2 tablespoons lemon zest
- 1/4 cup almond flour

Prep Time: 15 mins

Cooking Time: 25 mins

Total Time: 40 mins

Servings: 8

Nutrition Facts (per serving):

- Calories: 200
- Fat: 16g
- Saturated Fat: 5g
- Cholesterol: 85mg
- Sodium: 45mg
- Carbohydrate: 8g
- Protein: 7g
- Fiber: 3g

Directions:

1. Preheat oven to 350°F (175°C). Line an 8x8 inch baking pan with parchment paper.

2. Mix almond flour, erythritol, melted butter, and vanilla extract for the crust. Press evenly into the bottom of the prepared pan.

3. Bake the crust for 10 minutes, then remove from oven.

4. Whisk together eggs, erythritol, lemon juice, lemon zest, and almond flour for the filling. Pour over the pre-baked crust.

5. Return to oven and bake for an additional 15 minutes, or until the filling is set.

6. Cool completely before slicing into bars. Enjoy a tangy and sweet dessert that's perfect for a low-carb diet.

Coconut Flour Blueberry Muffins

Ingredients:

- 1/2 cup coconut flour
- 1/4 cup erythritol
- 1 teaspoon baking powder
- 1/4 teaspoon salt
- 6 eggs
- 1/2 cup coconut oil, melted
- 1/2 cup unsweetened almond milk
- 1 teaspoon vanilla extract
- 1 cup blueberries

Prep Time: 10 mins

Cooking Time: 20 mins

Total Time: 30 mins

Servings: 12

Nutrition Facts (per serving):

- Calories: 150
- Fat: 12g
- Saturated Fat: 9g
- Cholesterol: 85mg
- Sodium: 75mg
- Carbohydrate: 6g
- Protein: 4g
- Fiber: 3g

Directions:

1. Preheat oven to 350°F (175°C). Line a muffin tin with paper liners.
2. In a bowl, mix coconut flour, erythritol, baking powder, and salt.
3. In another bowl, whisk together eggs, melted coconut oil, almond milk, and vanilla extract.
4. Combine wet and dry ingredients until smooth. Gently fold in blueberries.
5. Divide batter among muffin cups and bake for 20 minutes, or until a toothpick inserted into the center comes out clean.
6. Serve as a delicious and nutritious breakfast option or snack, perfect for satisfying sweet cravings on a low-carb diet.

Raspberry Swirl Cheesecake

Ingredients:

For the crust:

- 1 cup almond flour
- 3 tablespoons butter, melted
- 1 tablespoon erythritol

For the filling:

- 16 oz cream cheese, softened
- 1/2 cup erythritol
- 2 eggs
- 1 teaspoon vanilla extract
- 1/2 cup raspberries, pureed

Prep Time: 20 mins

Cooking Time: 45 mins

Total Time: 1 hour 5 mins

Servings: 8

Nutrition Facts (per serving):

- Calories: 320
- Fat: 29g
- Saturated Fat: 16g
- Cholesterol: 125mg
- Sodium: 220mg
- Carbohydrate: 7g
- Protein: 7g
- Fiber: 2g

Directions:

1. Preheat oven to 325°F (165°C). Mix almond flour, melted butter, and erythritol for the crust. Press into the bottom of a springform pan.

2. Beat cream cheese and erythritol until smooth. Add eggs one at a time, then vanilla extract. Pour over the crust.

3. Dollop raspberry puree on top of the filling. Use a toothpick to swirl the puree into the filling.

4. Bake for 45 minutes, or until the edges are set but the center is slightly jiggly.

5. Cool, then refrigerate for at least 4 hours before serving. Enjoy a decadent and creamy dessert that's low in carbs and high in flavor.

Peanut Butter Chocolate Chip Cookies

Ingredients:

- 1 cup natural peanut butter
- 1/2 cup erythritol
- 1 egg
- 1/2 teaspoon baking soda
- 1/4 teaspoon salt
- 1/2 cup sugar-free chocolate chips

Prep Time: 10 mins

Cooking Time: 12 mins

Total Time: 22 mins

Servings: 12

Nutrition Facts (per serving):

- Calories: 180
- Fat: 14g
- Saturated Fat: 4g
- Cholesterol: 15mg
- Sodium: 200mg
- Carbohydrate: 8g
- Protein: 6g
- Fiber: 2g

Directions:

1. Preheat oven to 350°F (175°C). Line a baking sheet with parchment paper.

2. In a bowl, mix together peanut butter, erythritol, egg, baking soda, and salt until well combined. Stir in chocolate chips.

3. Scoop tablespoon-sized balls of dough onto the prepared baking sheet. Flatten slightly with a fork.

4. Bake for 12 minutes, or until the edges are golden but the centres are still soft.

5. Let cool on the baking sheet for 5 minutes, then transfer to a wire rack to cool completely. Enjoy a guilt-free treat that combines the classic flavours of peanut butter and chocolate.

Keto Chocolate Chip Cheesecake Bars

Ingredients:

For the crust:

- 1 cup almond flour

- 3 tablespoons unsalted butter, melted

- 1 tablespoon erythritol

For the filling:

- 16 oz cream cheese, softened

- 1/2 cup erythritol

- 2 large eggs

- 1 teaspoon vanilla extract

- 1/2 cup sugar-free chocolate chips

Prep Time: 15 mins

Cooking Time: 35 mins

Total Time: 50 mins

Servings: 12

Nutrition Facts (per serving):

- Calories: 280

- Fat: 25g

- Saturated Fat: 14g

- Cholesterol: 95mg

- Sodium: 180mg

- Carbohydrate: 6g

- Protein: 6g

- Fiber: 2g

Directions:

1. Preheat oven to 350°F (175°C). Line an 8x8 inch baking pan with parchment paper.

2. Combine almond flour, melted butter, and erythritol for the crust. Press evenly into the bottom of the prepared pan.

3. Beat cream cheese and erythritol until smooth. Add eggs one at a time, then vanilla extract. Fold in chocolate chips gently.

4. Pour the filling over the crust and smooth the top.

5. Bake for 35 minutes, or until the edges are set but the centre is slightly jiggly.

6. Cool completely, then refrigerate for at least 3 hours before cutting into bars. Enjoy a decadent, keto-friendly dessert that satisfies your sweet tooth.

Lemon Coconut Fat Bombs

Ingredients:

- 1 cup coconut oil, melted

- 1/2 cup unsweetened shredded coconut

- 1/4 cup fresh lemon juice

- Zest of 1 lemon, 2 tablespoons erythritol

Prep Time: 10 mins

Cooking Time: 0 mins

Total Time: 10 mins (plus freezing time)

Servings: 12

Nutrition Facts (per serving):

- Calories: 180

- Fat: 18g

- Saturated Fat: 16g

- Cholesterol: 0mg

- Sodium: 5mg

- Carbohydrate: 2g

- Protein: 1g

- Fiber: 1g

Directions:

1. In a bowl, mix together melted coconut oil, shredded coconut, lemon juice, lemon zest, and erythritol until well combined.

2. Pour the mixture into silicone molds or an ice cube tray.

3. Freeze until solid, about 1-2 hours.

4. Pop the fat bombs out of the molds and store in an airtight container in the freezer. Enjoy a refreshing and energizing keto snack that's perfect for a quick fat boost.

Strawberry Mascarpone Tart

Ingredients:

For the crust:

- 1 1/2 cups almond flour

- 1/4 cup unsalted butter, melted

- 1 tablespoon erythritol

For the filling:

- 8 oz mascarpone cheese, softened

- 1/4 cup erythritol

- 1 teaspoon vanilla extract

- 1 cup strawberries, sliced

Prep Time: 20 mins

Cooking Time: 10 mins

Total Time: 30 mins (plus chilling time)

Servings: 8

Nutrition Facts (per serving):

- Calories: 300

- Fat: 27g

- Saturated Fat: 12g

- Cholesterol: 55mg

- Sodium: 45mg

- Carbohydrate: 8g

- Protein: 6g

- Fiber: 3g

Directions:

1. Preheat oven to 350°F (175°C). Mix almond flour, melted butter, and erythritol for the crust. Press into a tart pan and bake for 10 minutes. Let cool.

2. Beat mascarpone cheese, erythritol, and vanilla extract until smooth. Spread over the cooled crust.

3. Arrange sliced strawberries on top of the filling.

4. Refrigerate for at least 2 hours before serving. Enjoy a luxurious and creamy dessert that's surprisingly simple to make and low in carbs.

No-Bake Peanut Butter Chocolate Bars

Ingredients:

- 1 cup natural peanut butter
- 1/2 cup coconut oil, melted
- 1/4 cup cocoa powder, 1/4 cup erythritol
- 1 teaspoon vanilla extract
- Pinch of salt

Prep Time: 10 mins

Cooking Time: 0 mins

Total Time: 10 mins (plus chilling time)

Servings: 12

Nutrition Facts (per serving):

- Calories: 220
- Fat: 20g
- Saturated Fat: 10g
- Cholesterol: 0mg
- Sodium: 100mg

- Carbohydrate: 6g

- Protein: 4g

- Fiber: 2g

Directions:

1. Line an 8x8 inch baking pan with parchment paper.

2. In a bowl, mix together peanut butter, melted coconut oil, cocoa powder, erythritol, vanilla extract, and a pinch of salt until smooth.

3. Pour the mixture into the prepared pan and smooth the top.

4. Freeze until solid, about 2 hours.

5. Cut into bars and serve. Store any leftovers in the freezer. Enjoy a rich and satisfying no-bake dessert that's perfect for chocolate and peanut butter lovers on a low-carb diet.

Cinnamon Roll Mug Cake

Ingredients:

- 2 tablespoons almond flour

- 1 tablespoon coconut flour

- 1 tablespoon erythritol

- 1/2 teaspoon baking powder

- 1/2 teaspoon cinnamon

- 1 egg

- 2 tablespoons unsweetened almond milk

- 1 tablespoon unsalted butter, melted

- 1/4 teaspoon vanilla extract

For the icing:

- 1 tablespoon cream cheese, softened

- 1 tablespoon erythritol

- 1/2 tablespoon unsweetened almond milk

Prep Time: 5 mins

Cooking Time: 2 mins

Total Time: 7 mins

Servings: 1

Nutrition Facts (per serving):

- Calories: 320

- Fat: 27g

- Saturated Fat: 12g

- Cholesterol: 215mg

- Sodium: 320mg

- Carbohydrate: 8g

- Protein: 10g

- Fiber: 3g

Directions:

1. In a microwave-safe mug, mix together almond flour, coconut flour, erythritol, baking powder, and cinnamon.

2. Stir in the egg, almond milk, melted butter, and vanilla extract until well combined.

3. Microwave on high for 90 seconds or until the cake is set.

4. For the icing, mix together softened cream cheese, erythritol, and almond milk until smooth. Drizzle over the warm mug cake.

5. Serve immediately for a quick and comforting dessert that's perfect for satisfying those cinnamon roll cravings without straying from a low-carb diet.

Keto Raspberry Swirl Cheesecake

Ingredients:

For the crust:

- 1 cup almond flour
- 3 tablespoons unsalted butter, melted
- 1 tablespoon erythritol

For the filling:

- 16 oz cream cheese, softened
- 3/4 cup erythritol
- 2 large eggs
- 1 teaspoon vanilla extract
- For the raspberry swirl:
- 1/2 cup raspberries
- 2 tablespoons erythritol

Prep Time: 20 mins

Cooking Time: 50 mins

Total Time: 1 hour 10 mins

Servings: 12

Nutrition Facts (per serving):

- Calories: 260
- Fat: 24g
- Saturated Fat: 13g
- Cholesterol: 95mg
- Sodium: 220mg
- Carbohydrate: 5g

- Protein: 6g

- Fiber: 1g

Directions:

1. Preheat oven to 325°F (165°C). Mix almond flour, melted butter, and erythritol for the crust. Press into the bottom of a springform pan and set aside.

2. Beat cream cheese and erythritol until smooth. Add eggs one at a time, then vanilla extract. Pour over the crust.

3. Blend raspberries and erythritol to make the raspberry swirl. Dollop on top of the filling and use a toothpick to create swirls.

4. Bake for 50 minutes, or until the edges are set but the centre is slightly jiggly. Cool, then refrigerate for at least 4 hours before serving. Enjoy a creamy cheesecake with a delightful raspberry swirl.

Chocolate Almond Keto Fudge

Ingredients:

- 1 cup almond butter

- 1/2 cup coconut oil

- 1/4 cup unsweetened cocoa powder

- 1/4 cup erythritol

- 1 teaspoon vanilla extract

- A pinch of salt

- 1/4 cup chopped almonds (for topping)

Prep Time: 10 mins

Cooking Time: 0 mins

Total Time: 10 mins (plus chilling time)

Servings: 16

Nutrition Facts (per serving):

- Calories: 180
- Fat: 16g
- Saturated Fat: 7g
- Cholesterol: 0mg
- Sodium: 5mg
- Carbohydrate: 4g
- Protein: 4g
- Fiber: 2g

Directions:

1. Melt almond butter and coconut oil together in a saucepan over low heat. Remove from heat.

2. Stir in cocoa powder, erythritol, vanilla extract, and a pinch of salt until smooth.

3. Pour the mixture into a lined 8x8 inch baking dish. Sprinkle chopped almonds on top.

4. Freeze until solid, about 2 hours. Cut into squares and serve. Store any leftovers in the refrigerator. Enjoy a rich and chocolatey keto-friendly fudge.

Lemon Poppy Seed Keto Muffins

Ingredients:

- 2 cups almond flour
- 1/2 cup erythritol
- 2 teaspoons baking powder
- 1/4 teaspoon salt

- 1/4 cup unsalted butter, melted
- 4 large eggs
- 1/3 cup unsweetened almond milk
- 2 tablespoons lemon juice
- Zest of 1 lemon
- 1 tablespoon poppy seeds

Prep Time: 10 mins

Cooking Time: 20 mins

Total Time: 30 mins

Servings: 12

Nutrition Facts (per serving):

- Calories: 190
- Fat: 17g
- Saturated Fat: 4g
- Cholesterol: 70mg
- Sodium: 105mg
- Carbohydrate: 5g
- Protein: 6g
- Fiber: 2g

Directions:

1. Preheat oven to 350°F (175°C). Line a muffin tin with paper liners.

2. Mix almond flour, erythritol, baking powder, and salt in a bowl.

3. In another bowl, whisk together melted butter, eggs, almond milk, lemon juice, and lemon zest.

4. Combine wet and dry ingredients, then fold in poppy seeds.

5. Divide batter among muffin cups and bake for 20 minutes, or until a toothpick inserted into the center comes out clean.

6. Serve as a delightful breakfast or snack, perfect for a low-carb diet.

Keto Berry Cobbler

Ingredients:

- 2 cups mixed berries (raspberries, blueberries, strawberries)
- 1 cup almond flour
- 1/4 cup erythritol
- 1/4 cup unsalted butter, melted
- 1 egg
- 1 teaspoon vanilla extract
- A pinch of salt

Prep Time: 10 mins

Cooking Time: 25 mins

Total Time: 35 mins

Servings: 8

Nutrition Facts (per serving):

- Calories: 180
- Fat: 15g
- Saturated Fat: 5g
- Cholesterol: 45mg
- Sodium: 55mg

- Carbohydrate: 7g

- Protein: 4g

- Fiber: 3g

Directions:

1. Preheat oven to 375°F (190°C). Place mixed berries in a greased 8x8 inch baking dish.

2. In a bowl, mix almond flour, erythritol, melted butter, egg, vanilla extract, and a pinch of salt until crumbly.

3. Sprinkle the mixture over the berries in the baking dish.

4. Bake for 25 minutes, or until the topping is golden and the berries are bubbly.

5. Serve warm, perhaps with a dollop of whipped cream. Enjoy a comforting and fruity dessert that fits perfectly into a keto lifestyle.

Keto Peanut Butter Cups

Ingredients:

- 1 cup sugar-free dark chocolate chips

- 1/2 cup natural peanut butter

- 1/4 cup coconut oil

- 2 tablespoons erythritol

- A pinch of salt

Prep Time: 15 mins

Cooking Time: 0 mins

Total Time: 15 mins (plus chilling time)

Servings: 12

Nutrition Facts (per serving):

- Calories: 150

- Fat: 13g

- Saturated Fat: 7g

- Cholesterol: 0mg

- Sodium: 75mg

- Carbohydrate: 6g

- Protein: 3g

- Fiber: 1g

Directions:

1. Melt half of the dark chocolate chips with half of the coconut oil in a microwave or double boiler. Stir until smooth.

2. Divide the melted chocolate among 12 muffin tin liners, placed in a muffin tin. Freeze for 10 minutes to set.

3. Mix peanut butter, erythritol, and a pinch of salt. Divide and spoon over the set chocolate base.

4. Melt the remaining chocolate chips and coconut oil, then spoon over the peanut butter layer.

5. Freeze until solid, about 1 hour. Enjoy a homemade version of the classic peanut butter cup that's keto-friendly and utterly delicious.

Keto Vanilla Bean Panna Cotta

Ingredients:

- 2 cups heavy cream

- 1 vanilla bean, split and seeds scraped

- 1/4 cup erythritol

- 1 teaspoon gelatin powder

- 1/4 cup water

- Fresh berries for garnish

Prep Time: 10 mins

Cooking Time: 5 mins

Total Time: 15 mins (plus chilling time)

Servings: 4

Nutrition Facts (per serving):

- Calories: 400

- Fat: 40g

- Saturated Fat: 25g

- Cholesterol: 150mg

- Sodium: 45mg

- Carbohydrate: 4g

- Protein: 2g

- Fiber: 0g

Directions:

1. In a small bowl, sprinkle gelatin over water and let it bloom for 5 minutes.

2. In a saucepan, combine heavy cream, erythritol, and the seeds from the vanilla bean. Heat over medium heat until it just begins to simmer. Remove from heat.

3. Add the bloomed gelatin to the cream mixture and stir until fully dissolved.

4. Pour the mixture into four serving glasses or ramekins. Refrigerate for at least 4 hours, or until set.

5. Serve garnished with fresh berries. Enjoy a creamy and luxurious dessert that's simple yet elegant, perfect for a keto-friendly treat.

Keto Matcha Green Tea Coconut Bars

Ingredients:

- 1 cup coconut butter, softened

- 1/2 cup coconut oil, melted

- 1/4 cup erythritol, 2 tablespoons matcha green tea powder

- 1 teaspoon vanilla extract

- Pinch of salt

- Unsweetened shredded coconut for topping

Prep Time: 10 mins

Cooking Time: 0 mins

Total Time: 10 mins (plus freezing time)

Servings: 12

Nutrition Facts (per serving):

- Calories: 220

- Fat: 22g

- Saturated Fat: 18g

- Cholesterol: 0mg

- Sodium: 25mg

- Carbohydrate: 4g

- Protein: 2g

- Fiber: 2g

Directions:

1. In a bowl, mix together coconut butter, coconut oil, erythritol, matcha powder, vanilla extract, and a pinch of salt until smooth.

2. Line an 8x8 inch baking dish with parchment paper and pour the mixture into the dish. Smooth the top with a spatula.

3. Sprinkle unsweetened shredded coconut over the top for added texture.

4. Freeze until solid, about 2 hours. Cut into bars and serve. Enjoy a refreshing and energizing treat that combines the unique flavor of matcha with the richness of coconut.

Keto Salted Caramel Mocha Mousse

Ingredients:

- 1 cup heavy cream
- 1/2 cup unsweetened cocoa powder
- 1/4 cup erythritol
- 2 tablespoons instant coffee granules
- 1 teaspoon vanilla extract
- 1/4 teaspoon sea salt
- Sugar-free caramel sauce for drizzling

Prep Time: 15 mins

Cooking Time: 0 mins

Total Time: 15 mins (plus chilling time)

Servings: 4

Nutrition Facts (per serving):

- Calories: 300
- Fat: 28g
- Saturated Fat: 17g

- Cholesterol: 100mg

- Sodium: 150mg

- Carbohydrate: 6g

- Protein: 3g

- Fiber: 2g

Directions:

1. In a large bowl, beat heavy cream until soft peaks form.

2. Gradually add cocoa powder, erythritol, instant coffee granules, vanilla extract, and sea salt, continuing to beat until well combined and stiff peaks form.

3. Spoon the mousse into serving dishes and refrigerate for at least 1 hour to set.

4. Before serving, drizzle with sugar-free caramel sauce and a sprinkle of sea salt. Enjoy a decadent and sophisticated dessert that perfectly balances the flavours of salted caramel and mocha.

Keto Lemon Ricotta Cake

Ingredients:

- 1 1/2 cups almond flour

- 3/4 cup erythritol

- 2 teaspoons baking powder

- 1/2 teaspoon salt

- 4 eggs

- 1 cup ricotta cheese

- 1/4 cup unsalted butter, melted

- Zest of 2 lemons

- 2 tablespoons lemon juice

- 1 teaspoon vanilla extract

Prep Time: 15 mins

Cooking Time: 35 mins

Total Time: 50 mins

Servings: 8

Nutrition Facts (per serving):

- Calories: 320

- Fat: 26g

- Saturated Fat: 10g

- Cholesterol: 135mg

- Sodium: 300mg

- Carbohydrate: 7g

- Protein: 12g

- Fiber: 3g

Directions:

1. Preheat oven to 350°F (175°C). Line an 8-inch round cake pan with parchment paper and grease the sides.

2. In a bowl, whisk together almond flour, erythritol, baking powder, and salt.

3. In another bowl, beat eggs, ricotta, melted butter, lemon zest, lemon juice, and vanilla extract until smooth.

4. Gradually add the dry ingredients to the wet ingredients, stirring until just combined.

5. Pour the batter into the prepared cake pan and smooth the top.

6. Bake for 35 minutes, or until a toothpick inserted into the centre comes out clean.

7. Let cool before serving. Enjoy a light and fluffy cake with a delightful lemon flavor, perfect for a keto-friendly dessert or afternoon tea.

Keto Chocolate Hazelnut Truffles

Ingredients:

- 1 cup hazelnuts, toasted and skins removed
- 3/4 cup heavy cream
- 1/2 cup sugar-free dark chocolate chips
- 1/4 cup unsweetened cocoa powder for coating
- 1/4 cup erythritol
- 1 teaspoon vanilla extract
- A pinch of salt

Prep Time: 20 mins

Cooking Time: 0 mins

Total Time: 20 mins (plus chilling time)

Servings: 12

Nutrition Facts (per serving):

- Calories: 180
- Fat: 16g
- Saturated Fat: 6g
- Cholesterol: 20mg
- Sodium: 20mg
- Carbohydrate: 6g
- Protein: 3g
- Fiber: 2g

Directions:

1. In a food processor, pulse hazelnuts until finely ground.

2. In a saucepan, heat heavy cream until it just begins to simmer. Remove from heat and add sugar-free dark chocolate chips, stirring until melted and smooth.

3. Stir in ground hazelnuts, erythritol, vanilla extract, and a pinch of salt into the chocolate mixture until well combined.

4. Refrigerate the mixture for at least 2 hours, or until firm enough to shape.

5. Using a spoon, scoop out portions of the mixture and roll into balls. Coat each truffle in unsweetened cocoa powder.

6. Store truffles in the refrigerator until ready to serve. Enjoy a rich and indulgent treat that's perfect for satisfying your sweet tooth on a keto diet.

28 DAY MEAL PLAN

Day 1:

- *Breakfast:* Lemon Poppy Seed Keto Muffins
- *Lunch:* Avocado and Egg Salad Cups
- *Dinner:* Zesty Lime and Shrimp Avocado Boats
- *Snack:* Keto Raspberry Swirl Cheesecake

Day 2:

- *Breakfast:* Keto Vanilla Bean Panna Cotta
- *Lunch:* Greek Salad Skewers
- *Dinner:* Keto Salted Caramel Mocha Mousse
- *Snack:* Cheesy Garlic Broccoli Bites

Day 3:

- *Breakfast:* Cinnamon Roll Mug Cake
- *Lunch:* Mini Pepperoni Pizza Bites
- *Dinner:* Lemon Coconut Fat Bombs
- *Snack:* Roasted Chickpeas with Rosemary and Sea Salt

Day 4:

- *Breakfast:* Keto Chocolate Avocado Pudding
- *Lunch:* Cheesy Stuffed Sweet Peppers
- *Dinner:* Keto Chocolate Chip Cheesecake Bars
- *Snack:* Bacon-Wrapped Avocado Fries

Day 5:

- *Breakfast:* Keto Matcha Green Tea Coconut Bars
- *Lunch:* Stuffed Jalapeño Poppers with Bacon and Cream Cheese

- *Dinner:* Keto Berry Cobbler
- *Snack:* Smoked Salmon Cucumber Bites

Day 6:

- *Breakfast:* Keto Peanut Butter Cups
- *Lunch:* Cucumber Shrimp Cocktail Cups
- *Dinner:* Keto Lemon Ricotta Cake
- *Snack:* Garlic Herb Roasted Nuts

Day 7:

- *Breakfast:* No-Bake Peanut Butter Chocolate Bars
- *Lunch:* Prosciutto and Melon Skewers
- *Dinner:* Strawberry Mascarpone Tart
- *Snack:* Chocolate Almond Keto Fudge

Day 8:

- *Breakfast:* Chocolate Almond Keto Fudge (leftovers)
- *Lunch:* Avocado Devilled Eggs
- *Dinner:* Keto Raspberry Swirl Cheesecake (leftovers)
- *Snack:* Cheesy Garlic Broccoli Bites (leftovers)

Day 9:

- *Breakfast:* Lemon Poppy Seed Keto Muffins (leftovers)
- *Lunch:* Greek Salad Skewers (leftovers)
- *Dinner:* Keto Salted Caramel Mocha Mousse (leftovers)
- *Snack:* Keto Peanut Butter Cups (leftovers)

Day 10:

- *Breakfast:* Cinnamon Roll Mug Cake (leftovers)

- *Lunch:* Mini Pepperoni Pizza Bites (leftovers)
- *Dinner:* Lemon Coconut Fat Bombs (leftovers)
- *Snack:* Roasted Chickpeas with Rosemary and Sea Salt (leftovers)

Day 11:

- *Breakfast:* Keto Chocolate Avocado Pudding
- *Lunch:* Stuffed Jalapeño Poppers with Bacon and Cream Cheese
- *Dinner:* Keto Lemon Ricotta Cake
- *Snack:* Garlic Herb Roasted Nuts

Day 12:

- *Breakfast:* Lemon Poppy Seed Keto Muffins
- *Lunch:* Greek Salad Skewers
- *Dinner:* Keto Berry Cobbler
- *Snack:* Cheesy Garlic Broccoli Bites

Day 13:

- *Breakfast:* Keto Vanilla Bean Panna Cotta
- *Lunch:* Avocado and Egg Salad Cups
- *Dinner:* Zesty Lime and Shrimp Avocado Boats
- *Snack:* Keto Raspberry Swirl Cheesecake

Day 14:

- *Breakfast:* Cinnamon Roll Mug Cake
- *Lunch:* Mini Pepperoni Pizza Bites
- *Dinner:* Keto Salted Caramel Mocha Mousse
- *Snack:* Bacon-Wrapped Avocado Fries

Day 15:

- *Breakfast:* Keto Matcha Green Tea Coconut Bars
- *Lunch:* Cheesy Stuffed Sweet Peppers
- *Dinner:* Keto Chocolate Chip Cheesecake Bars
- *Snack:* Smoked Salmon Cucumber Bites

Day 16:

- *Breakfast:* Keto Peanut Butter Cups
- *Lunch:* Cucumber Shrimp Cocktail Cups
- *Dinner:* Strawberry Mascarpone Tart
- *Snack:* Chocolate Almond Keto Fudge

Day 17:

- *Breakfast:* No-Bake Peanut Butter Chocolate Bars
- *Lunch:* Prosciutto and Melon Skewers
- *Dinner:* Lemon Coconut Fat Bombs
- *Snack:* Roasted Chickpeas with Rosemary and Sea Salt

Day 18:

- *Breakfast:* Keto Chocolate Avocado Pudding (leftovers)
- *Lunch:* Avocado Devilled Eggs
- *Dinner:* Keto Lemon Ricotta Cake (leftovers)
- *Snack:* Garlic Herb Roasted Nuts (leftovers)

Day 19:

- *Breakfast:* Lemon Poppy Seed Keto Muffins (leftovers)
- *Lunch:* Greek Salad Skewers (leftovers)
- *Dinner:* Keto Berry Cobbler (leftovers)

CONCLUSION

Our discussion focused on creating a comprehensive and varied meal plan tailored for individuals following a low-carb, keto-friendly diet. Over the course of 30 days, we outlined a series of meal plans that incorporate a wide range of recipes designed to satisfy different tastes and preferences while adhering to the nutritional guidelines of a ketogenic lifestyle. Each plan was carefully constructed to ensure variety, with a mix of savoury and sweet options, and included breakfast, lunch, dinner, and snack suggestions.

The recipes provided were selected for their nutritional value, ease of preparation, and compatibility with a low-carb diet. From hearty breakfast options like Lemon Poppy Seed Keto Muffins to satisfying dinners such as Keto Salted Caramel Mocha Mousse and snacks like Garlic Herb Roasted Nuts, the meal plans aimed to offer delicious and nutritious choices for every part of the day. Desserts were not overlooked, with options like Keto Raspberry Swirl Cheesecake and Keto Chocolate Chip Cheesecake Bars allowing for indulgence without deviating from dietary goals.

Key to the success of these meal plans is their flexibility. We emphasized the importance of adjusting portion sizes to individual dietary needs and preferences, as well as the option to swap meals between days for convenience and variety. The inclusion of fresh, non-starchy vegetables and the recommendation to stay hydrated were also highlighted as essential components of a balanced keto diet.

www.ingramcontent.com/pod-product-compliance
Lightning Source LLC
Chambersburg PA
CBHW051605250726
48653CB00004BA/1334